Six Weeks to a Healthy Lifestyle

Six Weeks to a Healthy Lifestyle

Betty Sue O'Brian

Betty O'Brian is a Traditional Naturopath who focuses upon helping others to understand the truth about healthy living.

For more information about her speeches, workshops, and trainings, contact her at betty.obrian@gmail.com or 228-257-1946. Visit her websites: bettysueobrian.com and iridologyacademy.org.

First published in 2008;

2nd edition 2010, 2015

3rd edition 2017

O'Brian, Betty.

Six weeks to a healthy lifestyle

1. Health and Wellbeing

Cover design by Mary Rowe and Melissa Sutherland
Cover photographs by Mary Rowe and Melissa Sutherland
Edited by Jackie Parker

ISBN 978-1-5151-1928-9

Printed in the United States of America

With love and gratitude

For the magnitude of his faith

And the power of his calm inner spirit,

I dedicate this book to my husband, John Duke Sutherland.

Table of Contents

Clean up your body... Clean up your Home... Clean up your Life

Beware, as you go through this six-week program, you just might clean up the garage and the attic along with your body!

Foreword

I clearly remember the first time that I met Betty Sue O'Brian.

It was at a health conference in Las Vegas, Nevada, some years ago, I was extremely impressed with this soft spoken, distinguished looking professor from Mississippi and her willingness to step outside the so-called "box" in so many different areas of her life. Often, I find those who are entrenched in academia somewhat resistant to change or new ideas, but as I came to know Betty Sue, that was certainly not true of her. I've found her to be passionate about learning new things and just as passionate about teaching these new ideas to others. She is an excellent student, takes what she learns to the level of mastery and becomes the master teacher.

It's a tragedy that, in a nation that spends more on health care than any other nation, over 70% of us are overweight. Arthritis, osteoporosis, cancer, diabetes, heart disease, mental illness and many other conditions are running rampant in America. Most of us have loved ones suffering from these and other terrible maladies that are preventable if we just understood the real underlying cause and what to do to prevent them.

To make matters worse, we are leading our young people down the same path only at a much-accelerated rate. Children in America are experiencing diseases earlier in life than they've ever occurred in previous generations, and drug companies have found America's youth to be an incredible new market for their drugs, starting them younger and younger on these dangerous prescription medications with so many negative side-effects.

The truth is that doing what we're doing hasn't been working for Americans, and it's time for a change. I've watched thousands and thousands of people change their lives by following the correct principles of health that are taught by Betty Sue in this book. I've watched the miracles as they get their health back, from high blood pressure to high cholesterol, from obesity to diabetes, from arthritis and joint pain to chronic fatigue and fibromyalgia. I know that this works!

I've taught my patients that everything in life is about balance. If we think about the teeter-totters we played on in grade school, we will remember that as long as the person sitting on the other end from us was approximately the same weight, things went pretty well, but when they were twice our size we were constantly high in the air and getting bumped around a lot. Our bodies work in the same way, and as long as we stay in the "healthy zone" of balance, we do fine, but if we get out of balance in one or two areas in our lives, we'll find ourselves being sick.

True health empowers us to be all that we can be and to achieve our Life's Purpose with all of our physical, spiritual and mental abilities operating efficiently and in harmony. Without this health and vitality, we spend most of our time in survival mode, usually just treating symptoms and not the underlying causes, which usually means that we really don't get better. And with all of the special-interest groups out there advertising their products, it's very easy to get confused about what to do and what really works. In this wonderful book, Betty Sue teaches us how to take this amazing body of ours (I call it the Billion Dollar Machine because it's so amazing) and help it work optimally by teaching the true fundamentals of health.

Betty Sue is a world-class teacher, who can take complicated ideas and subjects and teach them to anyone at their level of learning. In this wonderful book, she helps teach us the fundamentals of health, which then empowers us to have the energy and vitality to live our lives to the fullest. Do yourself a big favor and read this book, then apply what you learn to your life for 90 days and experience the true health and vitality that you've been missing in your life!

-Dave Carpenter, N.D., C. Ac., C.C.I and owner of Path to Health, LLC

Introduction

We are all connected. We are all connected, not only with all humanity, but also with all there is. As our world influences us, we in turn influence our world. Yet, for 100 years as we have migrated away from the land, we have lost much of the knowledge that our mother's mother took for granted. As factory farms and long-distance transportation have replaced the monthly trip to the market, pharmaceutical companies and chemical manufacturers have replaced a common knowledge of plants and herbs ... and common sense. My grandmother found her chicken in the yard. My mother found her chicken wrapped in plastic in the grocery. I find my chicken grown locally, free-range and organic. We have moved far away from the sources of our sustenance, and we can't all go back to the land, but I believe we can turn the corner and regain balance and find a more natural harmony on Earth, one choice at a time.

Originally, I wrote this book to give others a glimpse into the worlds of herbs, chakras, natural health, cleansing, vegetarianism, and the alkaline lifestyle. The course has become, for most who take it, a step-by-step guide and a life-changing education. People used to smoke in stores and offices, putting out cigarettes on the concrete floors of grocery stores and lighting up in reading sections of libraries. Today we are appalled at the suggestion. A major shift occurred. My vision for the United States is of a country where everyone can get organic foods, where herbs are the preferred remedy for illness as well as for the promotion of health, and where the lesson that "giving really is receiving" is accepted by all.

Today even the average American is looking at the chemical content of foods: the state of New York has outlawed trans-fats in restaurants; Wal-Mart is developing its organic products, and medical doctors are joining the forces of herbalists and using complimentary healing modalities. There has been a paradigm shift, and change is happening quickly. We even have icons of health in the medical profession: Dr. Andre Rocco, Dr. Andrew Weill, Dr. Deepak Chopra, Dr. Mehmet Oz and hundreds of others trained in natural living by these amazing integrative physicians. My concern is for the person who wants to use natural means to heal or to build health; he or she needs guidance from an informed professional. Often, people enter the little office where I work as a naturopathic physician with medicines from the pharmacy and a bag full of supplements from various sources; sometimes they are feeling worse than before they started their healing journey.

Sometimes the solution is as simple as knowing about the soy-hypothyroid link when someone consumes soy for a long time. Certain cruciferous vegetables belonging to the cabbage family contain goitrogens, which are thyroid suppressants. Soy and foods such as tofu and veggie burgers and vegetables such as broccoli, cauliflower, turnips, and cabbage provide great nutrition but also can block thyroid function in certain people who are sensitive to them and have thyroid problems. Just adding some correct food choices such as natural kelp or natural barley greens can raise the level of a sluggish thyroid gland. Sometimes nutritional support and certain inversion yoga postures (shoulder and head stands) might help the situation, but how many people are able to figure out this sort of problem with just a knowledge of health and nutrition learned from magazines, TV or the internet?

Others are trying to lose weight by eating "no fat" and "low fat" crackers, cookies, yogurt, etc., and not understanding how the body thrives on good fats and suffers without them. Young women are developing candida and other yeast from an overload of sugar and hydrogenated fats found in most processed foods, especially low fat ones. Their poor little cells hold on tight to the water and fats they are allowed, leaving them feeling bloated and uncomfortable and not a bit lighter. As they continue eating low fat and high protein, consuming more Diet Coke and Splenda as they go, they get fatter rather than thinner. Their tissues become more inflamed and more acidic, creating an inner environment that promotes cellular changes and leads to further illnesses.

On a similar path, the organs get stripped away one by one – first the tonsils and adenoids, then the appendix or uterus. Next goes the gallbladder. With each procedure come more antibiotics, causing these "patients" to lose the wonderful, beneficial bacteria required by the human body. Harmful microorganisms love this acidic environment and begin to crowd out our helpful bacteria, destroying other tissues. They clamor for more sugar, more protein, more yeast, and they don't quiet down until we feed them. This lasts a short while as the intestines fill with gas, and reflux begins to burn the esophagus - not a pretty picture.

Then there are the prescription meds to suppress natural processes: put out the fires of digestion with the purple pill, add pancreatic enzymes, take a pill to force peristaltic action in the colon, swallow laxatives which pull needed water from the cells and tissues, leaving dehydration and inflammation behind.

Could asthma and emphysema be treated by destroying yeast, molds and bacteria, restoring balance in the lungs?

Could digestive issues really be solved by cleaning the intestines and toning, making simple dietary changes and drinking more high-quality, alkaline water?

What about the diabetes epidemic among adults and children? Could Dr. Young (PH Miracle) and Dr. Barody (Alkalize or Die) be right about acidity being the cause of so many chronic diseases such as diabetes? Will alkalizing the diet be enough to balance insulin usage and production in a type 2 diabetic?

What about cholesterol and the side effects of cholesterol lowering, statin drugs? Is the cholesterol scare in this country true, or do we need to discern what is making the cholesterol go up and "treat" it with fewer acids in our diet, B Vitamins, policosanol (from sugar cane), Omega 3's, and other good fats and oils?

Are our homes one of the sources of many of our illnesses? Xenoestrogens, found in man-made products such as Carpet Fresh and Pine Sol, flood our indoor environments and therefore our bodies. New carpet, blinds, and polyurethane coatings exude harmful artificial estrogens into the home air. How can we avoid their harmful effects short of moving to the deep woods or the desert?

Consider not only where we live and what we eat, but also what we apply to the hair, teeth and skin. Imagine that everything we put on our bodies is absorbed and enters the bloodstream to be handled and eliminated by the lymph. The fluoride and sodium laurel sulfate in toothpaste and aluminum in antiperspirants go into the body. Doesn't a warning not to swallow what you brush your teeth with seem like a red flag to you?

I was speaking to my vet about my dog's diet. She suggested that the indoor environment and the commercial food might be the reason for his skin problems and lethargy. "Put him on this organic, natural food with omega threes... and take him outside as much as possible." Has your doctor ever advised you to consider these factors in your own health? The vet knows that the hormones and pesticides might be harming the pets, yet humans are drinking milk from cows that have been shot full of hormones and fed on genetically engineered grains to fatten them up. Then the milk is homogenized and pasteurized to be sure that nothing could live in it, not even the good bacteria necessary for digestion and absorption of nutrients.

How important are emotions in the creation of illness and disease? What part do emotional patterns play in the inheritance of illness? Patterns of anger, hatred, resentment, and jealousy; do they stress us to the point of physical manifestation and breakdown, and is there a way to break these patterns in this lifetime so that our children do not have to inherit them? When the Bible says that the sins of the fathers are visited upon the children up to four generations, does it refer to these patterns that go deep into the physical and emotional body and create illness. In a family, there might be a pattern of anger in the fathers or poor communications, or a pattern of negativity or criticism.

In her books, *The Creation of Health* and *The Anatomy of the Spirit*, Carolyn Myss shows how belief patterns begin to manifest in the body. Cancer relates to the pattern of resentment, and pancreatitis and diabetes often follow the loss of the "sweetness of life."

This little book tries to address the questions above. Taking care of ourselves "as God intended" demonstrates to us and to God that we are serious about making changes in ourselves and in our world.

When I was a teenager, we often said, with hope, "Lighting one little candle makes the world a better place." This class is about lighting your candle, increasing white light around you as everyone in contact with you "catches" the light. Live longer, live more, love more, and "When you follow your bliss ... doors will open where you would not have thought there would be doors and where there wouldn't be a door for anyone else."[1]

---

[1] Campbell, Joseph. *Transformations of Myth Through Time.*

How To Use This Book

"Man... sacrifices his health in order to make money. Then he sacrifices money to recuperate his health. And then he is so anxious about the future that he does not enjoy the present; the result being that he does not live in the present or the future; he lives as if he is never going to die, and then dies having never really lived." - Daila Lama

Congratulations on reading this book and Taking Steps towards your improving your health! Each chapter is focused on a different aspect of how you can help yourself (and your family). At the end of each chapter, you can decide what specific steps you are going to take immediately.

One of the most important ideas throughout the book is the awareness that we need to put **acid on the outside** (skin) and **alkaline on the inside** (diet). This won't make sense to you until you read and learn more, but we will keep coming back to it.

Don't expect to take all the steps at once because of the amount of change and because of the cost of taking some steps such as replacing all of your lotions and cosmetics, and buying new products. But keep coming back to this book as you learn and grow, and are ready for more steps. You can also use this book to provide gift ideas to others! Tell your friends that you want a Neti pot for your birthday! Or put your soap, shampoo and lotions in the guest bathroom and buy some organic products for your body!

There is so much information available today that it can be confusing and sometimes misleading, but visit the Taking Steps website to learn more and to get your questions answered; join us at TakeStepsToHealth.com.

We encourage you to write your intentions on the pages of this book, turn the corners, and highlight the ideas that catch your attention! Use it as a workbook.

Week One: Take Steps to Care for Your Body!

"The greatest wealth is health." ~Virgil

A recent commercial on TV featured a youthful-looking, older woman who said "When you have got your health, you have just about everything." Anyone who has been sick for just a little while knows the significance of that statement. How many rich and famous would trade their moment of fame to reclaim their health.

Each of us is doing things each day that are health defeating rather than health promoting, and we often fret out loud about eating better and exercising more. People know they need to improve the diet... but what if they could feel better just by changing their personal beauty routine?

Probably the biggest complaint I hear in my office is, "I just don't have any energy; I'm tired." Where do you begin when you are feeling depleted – your hair is lifeless, the skin has rashes and blemishes, and your fingernails are breaking off. Do you want more energy? How would you like to get off of some medications by just changing your personal beauty routine? Most people want to feel better and have more vitality, but they lack the time to revamp their lives. Making time for massages and yoga and walking is one of the best things you can do for yourself, but let's assume you want to start cleaning up your physical body just by taking away the items in your kitchen and bath that might be creating problems for your health.

The skin is the largest organ of the body and absorbs everything; would you swallow your shampoo, put Victoria's Secret hand lotion on your heart or liver, or inject artificially scented and colored body soap into your kidneys? No, but your body must deal with the chemicals in every lotion, shampoo, and antiperspirant.

1

Trans-dermal patches for quitting smoking or balancing hormones demonstrate how effective the skin is as an uptake receptor, yet we apply toxic after shaves, hair dyes, and hair removal chemicals routinely. The skin, a secondary organ of elimination, mirrors our overall health and well-being. You can care for your skin, body, hair and nails by adopting some of the following more natural products and techniques.

Your Goals

Here is a summary of the best ways for you to take care of your skin, eyes, mouth, hair and nails. We will get into the details in the next pages. Your goal is to make all of these changes eventually. Do you do any of these already?

Skin Care:

- ☐ Apply only natural products to the skin

- ☐ Bathe in salts, oils, and clays

- ☐ Brush to stimulate the lymph and skin with a natural bristle brush

- ☐ Use natural salves for blemishes and skin cancer

- ☐ Use only crystals or aluminum-free deodorants for underarm care

Eyes and Sinus Care:

- ☐ Support the eyes and sinuses with herbs, a Neti pot, colloidal silver, and ear candling

- ☐ Use eyebright rinses to support the eye structure

Mouth Care:

- ☐ Avoid chemicals such as fluoride and sodium laurel sulfate in toothpastes

- ☐ Use mercury-free dentistry

☐ Use natural solutions for mouth, tooth and gum issues such as natural essential oil rinses

☐ Invest in an Ionic or sonic (Sonicare or Oral B) toothbrush

Hair and Nails Care:

☐ Support with all-natural herbal shampoos and natural henna rinses

☐ Treat nail infections and fungus with oregano and tea tree essential oil

Best Practices for the Skin

Tip 1 - Natural Skin Care

Use only natural skin care products that you make yourself or purchase from an organic source; consider some of the following for daily skin care.

Apple Cider Vinegar and Lemon Juice – Women in traditional cultures put food on their face. In the morning, make a large glass of lemon water with cayenne to drink. Squeeze the extra lemon on the backs of your hands and rub some on the face; watch the age spots fade away! Carry a small bottle of vinegar in your purse to soften and clean the hands after shopping or at work. Be sure to use organic apple cider vinegar with the 'mother' in them, because these are living foods with an active ingredient, e.g. Braggs.

Extra Virgin Coconut Oil – Use on the entire body. In addition to the products formulated just for skin care, just enjoy Extra Virgin Coconut Oil applied like a lotion. Coconut oil contains caprylic acid which is known to destroy yeast and fungus on the skin. Coconut oil has a wonderful scent all its own, but mixed with essential oils of lavender, sandalwood, orange, frankincense, etc., it becomes heavenly. This oil soaks into the skin readily and leaves it feeling soft and nourished, and it works beautifully for removing make up. Of course, you can eat it, too, which is always a good trait for anything put on the body.

French Green Cosmetic Clay - French green clay is also known as Sea Clay and is one of the most widely used for facial masks. The clay gets a green color from naturally decomposed plants and iron oxides. The molecular makeup of the clay is absorbent to the skin. Apply the clay to the skin in a smooth paste and enjoy the effect of toxins being drawn out of the skin. After a clay mask, you will be left with baby-soft skin.

Tropical Tradition Moisturizing Cream or Lotion and Exfoliating Salts – These products are pure and are in a base of extra virgin coconut oil and essential oils without any harsh chemicals.

Triple C Cream – A beautiful blend of three flowers; calendula, comfrey, and coneflower. This cream builds and restores tissue and makes a wonderful cream for diaper rash, scrapes and cuts. Some use it as a night cream for the face and hands, too.

Tip 2- Skin Brushing

Stimulate and exfoliate the skin by brushing daily with a natural bristle brush. The skin is known as the 3rd kidney, along with the lungs, and if it is clogged with hidden, poisonous waste, the body won't receive the nourishment it needs; nor will it be able to dispel toxins through this vital eliminative organ. After skin brushing, the skin feels alive and well and ready to meet the day.

Natural-bristle skin brushes are now available at stores like Bed, Bath and Beyond and Target. Get a long-handled brush so you can reach down your back, and pick up some organic olive oil, extra virgin coconut oil or jojoba oil.

This is what you do!

- Brush **before** showering or bathing when the skin is dry, not wet, for better exfoliation.

- Always brush **towards** the heart

  o Brush downwards on your face and neck.

  o Brush the palms of the hands, the backs of the hands and then up the arms.

  o Brush the feet and up the legs, always brushing towards the heart, then brush the back.

  o Go counter clockwise on the abdomen and use lighter strokes over and around the breasts.

- Oil the skin **before** you get into a bath or shower.

- Start the water as cold as you can in order to close the pores and absorb the good oils you have applied. It will also wake when and where you really need to. Let the oil soak into and feed your skin.

- The brush will easily hang outside the shower curtain on one of the shower curtain rings. Occasionally clean the bristle brush with warm, soapy water (natural soap, of course). Put in the sun to dry.

Tip 3- Bathing

Use bathing to rejuvenate the body. Try some of the following therapeutic bathing experiences.

Epsom Salts: What's so great about salt bathing? When magnesium sulfate (Epsom Salt) is absorbed through the skin, such as in a bath, it actually pulls toxins from the body, relaxes the nervous system, reduces inflammation, relaxes muscles, and exfoliates the skin. Run a warm bath and add two to four cups of Epsom salts; give it a little time to dissolve before you get in and relax for twenty minutes or more. Ahhh…

Clay Baths: Clay masks and clay body packs have the power to draw and pull toxins out of the body. Lauana Lei's says that a clay bath… "Pulls Pollutants Out Like A Magnet".[2] While the bath clean-up can be a bit tricky, the alkalizing, drawing properties of clay are worth the effort; use bentonite clay water for colon cleansing to draw toxins out of the lining of the intestines.

Foot Soak: Not only will it soften the skin, it will even exfoliate and clean, removing odors along with it and improving toenail problems such as fungus. Add 1/2 cup of Epsom Salts to a large pan of warm water. Soak feet for at least 30 minutes for the best benefit. My mother used Epsom Salts for sprains and infections as well. To multiply the benefits, try ionic footbaths to balance the body, regulate yeast and parasites, and speed up the cleansing and healing process. An ionic footbath produces negative ions electrically, similar to an ionic air cleaner. These ions attach to positive ions in the body and help to balance the electrical system.

Skin Exfoliator: Rub handfuls of Dead Sea or Celtic Sea Salts that have been scented with essential oils – Rosemary (invigorating), Lavender (calming), Peppermint (stimulating), etc. all over the body. Then shower. This treatment is a little scratchy the first time you do it to yourself, but it is very stimulating to the skin and helps to eliminate toxins and clear up skin eruptions.

Minerals and salts make the bath water feel silky and leave skin cleansed and soft. Here is a formula that you can make for yourself:

---

[2] Lei, Lauana. Magnetic Clay Baths.

Basic Salt Soak Bath Formula

1 cup sea salts (e.g. Himalayan sea salt, Celtic salt)

1 cup baking soda

1 cup Epsom salts

Combine the sea salts, baking soda, and Epsom salts in a bowl. Stir to blend. Pour 1/4 cup or so into the bath while the tub is filling. Some people add 1 to 2 tablespoons jojoba and essential oils to keep the skin from drying out (more for dry skin, less for oily.)

Tip 4 – Skin Relief:

For **Burns and Sunburns**, rub 2 Tbsp. Aloe Vera gel (or the amount from one leaf of the aloe vera plant) on the affected area several times immediately after being burned. Add 5 drops lavender essential oil to the 2 Tbsp. Aloe Vera gel; mix the two together and put directly on the burned skin. Acidic water from an ionizer definitely relieves sunburns and dry, itchy skin.

For **kitchen burns**, it is best to use powdered Vitamin C (ascorbic acid) directly on the burn. First moisten the hand or burned area; gently rub the Vitamin C on and leave it as a poultice. Vitamin C is a must for every kitchen!

Since we are talking about the sun here, **get your 15 minutes of sunshine** each day to get all the vitamin D that you need. Vitamin D promotes calcium absorption in the gut and moves calcium across cell membranes, making both the nervous and skeletal systems stronger. It also helps to stimulate the pineal gland and regulates the production of melatonin. In the book, *Love Without End: Jesus Speaks*, Glenda Green writes, "However, don't forget what I told you about sunlight; to watch the sun in the morning and the evening, because watching the sun can set your physical, ethereal, and spiritual hearts into a harmonic resonance which will attract what you need and process what you have more perfectly"

People suffering from auto-immune diseases such as multiple sclerosis and Crohn's disease are often low in vitamin D. Lab experiments show that vitamin D can also prevent the growth and spread of tumors, so don't forget about sunshine: it just might cheer you up as well.

Skin moles, skin tags, skin cancers: Rubbing extra virgin coconut oil on the skin after bathing is the place to start; the caprylic acid in the oils will soothe and calm the skin and make some eruptions disappear. Use Poke Salve made from the poke leaf or castor oil on the skin for minor skin eruptions.

Deeper skin problems may require the use of Black Salve or C Cream, but be sure to work with someone who knows what they are doing. These powerful drawing salves contain bloodroot and other strong herbs which have been known to eliminate many skin problems without surgery. Long used by American Indians, its rise is questioned by traditional medicine today, but I've seen (and had) amazing results from its use. Contact me for information on ordering or order through www.takestepstohealth.com.

Best Practices for the Eyes, Sinus and Ears

Tip 1- Eye and Sinus Care

Eyebright tincture – rinse the eyes daily with an eye cup and several drops of Dr. Christopher's Eyebright formula mixed with clean water. Dr. Christopher, 20th century American herbalist who created over fifty formulas still used today, claims that this formula nourishes the eyes and will even dissolve corneal signs. Lower your head, press the eye cup to your open eye, and tilt your head backwards.

Neti Pot – This little pot cleans and clears the sinus cavity by irrigation. It looks like a tea pot with a long spout. You fill it with salt water to cleanse the sinus and (this needs an explanation of what to do). If you have an infection, you can add a couple drops of Goldenseal or Colloidal silver. Keeping the sinuses clean with this little pot will help even the most chronic sinus conditions.

Ear Candling – Ear candles are hollow candles made of beeswax or paraffin; use them in the ears and on the body.

In the ears, the smoke from the candle heats the ear canal; as blood rushes to the area to cool, excess wax is pulled out by the smoke, providing better hearing and relieving pressure. Follow the instructions on the packet but basically you lay on your side, insert the ear candle, and let it burn down. If you are nervous, do this with a friend for the first time.

If the candle is placed directly on the skin where the infection is, it helps to relieve pain and infection – a very inexpensive and harmless cure that might be effective in many cases. My husband once had an infected tooth that the dentist said had to have a root canal, but after four ear candles on the jaw and on the gum, he was pain free. It is now six years later, and the tooth is still there. Since then, we have had several similar success stories with the teeth.

I have also used immune-building herbal supplements such as Elderberry, Echinacea, and Arabinogalactin, to assist with the clearing the infection. With the candling and the herbs, you'll have a better chance at healing naturally.

Tip 2- Tooth and Mouth Care

Read the label on your toothpaste. The word "natural" seems to be appearing on everything these days, but just because a toothpaste says natural ... well. You know that marketing ploy by now.

Avoid tooth products with fluoride and chemicals such as sodium laurel sulfate and unrecognizable names followed by numbers; these should make you very suspicious. Remember, those chemicals that go into your mouth will be absorbed into your body. Did you know that Colgate and other major brands have this warning on the back? "Keep out of the reach of children under 6. If more than used for brushing is accidentally swallowed, get medical help or contact a Poison Control Center"

Look for products with Neem, Tea Tree oil, and all herbal ingredients. A wonderful toothpaste made by Tropical Traditions is made from coconut oil.

Peppermint oil and tea tree oil mixed with water and food-grade peroxide clean the mouth well. Plain sea salt or baking soda mixed with food-grade peroxide[3] is great for the gums and teeth. Brush with baking soda and food- grade peroxide. Put a drop of peppermint and/or Tea Tree essential oils right onto the toothbrush.

Most of us put the toothbrush near the toilet on the bathroom sink; one can imagine the bacteria. **Clean toothbrushes** in food-grade peroxide weekly. Make a practice of replacing your toothbrush on the first of every month; as the month changes, it will occur to you to replace your toothbrush.

Scrape the tongue every morning with the back of a spoon or a metal tongue scraper to remove lymphatic waste.

Invest in a simple **ionic toothbrush**; ionic brushes use a negative ion to better attract the plaque which has a positive charge.

Holistic dentists say that **there is no safe root canal**; get a second opinion from a dentist familiar with the work of Westin Price and Hal Huggins. Use mercury-free dentistry, and avoid sealants for children and adults. Investigate the chemicals applied; some studies show that they leach bisphenol-A (BPA), an endocrine disruptor, so without a strong family history of dental decay, you might want to avoid them. Also, if the sealant is not applied extremely well, it can

---

[3] Food-grade peroxide is 3% strength; not the one in most grocery and drug stores.

actually lead to very serious cavities under the seal which are much harder to detect.

Tip 3 - Mouth Treatments

For an effective **mouth disinfectant**, add 3 to 4 drops of tincture of myrrh or a drop or two of tea tree or myrrh essential oil to a glass of water. Swish in mouth for one minute.

Clove oil is a safe remedy for **toothache**; it is a wonderful anesthetic for painful gums; you'll have excellent results with putting a few whole cloves on either side of the painful area. Hold FOOD GRADE peroxide (3%) diluted with water in the mouth for five minutes while showering. Swish around the teeth. This cleans the mouth and brightens the teeth.

Find and buy some Essential Herb Cottage Tooth Tonic —This tonic includes bloodroot and goldenseal to draw toxins from cavities where teeth have been pulled. It also provides amazing relief for any disturbances such as abscesses and irritations of the teeth or gums.

Make your own mouthwash with FOOD GRADE (3%) peroxide, water, and essential oil of wintergreen and tea tree oil or one drop of basil, oregano and peppermint. 1/3 reconstituted peroxide, 2/3 distilled water, and essential oils.

You can also use a drop of grapefruit seed extract; it is very bitter but disinfects the mouth and can be applied directly to an aching tooth.

For **Bleeding gums**, rinse and swish colloidal silver and/or liquid minerals in the mouth to disinfect and re-mineralize. A proven method is to follow this protocol:

- Switch to a neem/tea tree oil toothpaste

11

- Swish twice daily with colloidal minerals to re-mineralize the tissues and strengthen tooth enamel

- Take goldenseal for two weeks on and two weeks off for a few months

- Try baking soda and peroxide mixed for an occasional deep cleaning of the gums

Does your dog have bad breath? Put some drops of Colloidal silver into the water bowl every day. This will kill the bacteria in the mouth and prevent tooth decay.

Tip 4 - Hair Care

Anything that you put onto your scalp, will be absorbed into your body, so read the labels on your hair care products.

Watch for ingredients such as methyl paraben and sodium lauryl sulfate. Although it has not been proven to be harmful, sodium lauryl sulfate is the main ingredient in some concrete floor cleaners, so is it really appropriate for your skin?[4]

Often its presence in a shampoo or other skin care product may indicate other undesirable ingredients, such as formaldehyde preservatives or possible cancer-causing wetting agents such as DEA and nitrosamine-forming agents. According to Michael Wrightson, president of Logona Kosmetik, Germany is making a concerted effort to label personal products as certified natural, and in Germany, sodium lauryl sulfate, ammonium lauryl sulfate or sodium lauryl sulfate

---

[4] Weill, Andrew, M.D. www.drweill.com. Accessed March 6, 2008.

will prevent a product from being certified natural.[5]

You will have no trouble finding natural products. Use Giovanni and Aubry Organics and Dr. Bronner's Castile soaps—peppermint, lavender, almond and eucalyptus scented—for a healthy, clean scent. Visit the websites for Desert Essence and NOW.

If you want to "wash those chemicals right out of your hair" then make a vinegar rinse– Mix 1 part organic cider vinegar in 2 parts water and use it as an after-rinse to remove build-up of shampoos and conditioners.

Henna nourishes hair and is available in all colors; it's not just red anymore! Natural hair colorings are available now, as more and more companies answer our demands for safer hair color.

When I started to get grey, I went to the hair salon for color. My scalp burned each time I went and was red and tender for days. When I switched to Herbatint (from Italy) at the urging of a European friend, all discomfort associated with hair color ended, and my hair color lasted as long as it had with the more toxic salon color. Finally, I just stayed grey! It is better for my body, much cheaper, and I have decided to age gracefully and naturally.

Tip 5 - Nail Infections

Fingernail or toenail infections may be fungal and can indicate systemic yeast. They are often quite difficult to treat. People are more susceptible to fungal infections if they have a weakened immune system, diabetes, or a history of athlete's foot. Also, coats of toenail polish actually prevent the nail from breathing

---

[5] Wrightson, Michael. Aubrey Organics. www.aubrey- organics.com/about/articles. Accessed December 1, 2007.

and promote the growth of fungus. Painting on a commercial cure from the local drug store is not a permanent solution!

The problems with the drug therapies such as Sporanox include side effects such as nausea, headaches, insomnia, confusion, vomiting, dizziness, fatigue, and even liver damage! Plus, the patient has to take the drugs for three or more months, and the cure is not a guarantee. Are these side effects worth it if you could just perform a natural treatment first?

These problems should be treated both internally by taking supplements and externally by soaking the nail.

Internally, boost your immune system by taking capsules or drops of echinacea, cat's claw, elderberry, astragalus, arabinogalactan and eat shitake mushrooms. You can take any other immune supporting herbal formulas[6].

Externally, trim the nail back as far as you can and then try one of these two approaches.

Apply oil of oregano and tea tree oil with a Q-tip or soft toothbrush once or twice a day, but especially after bathing. Be careful because oregano may irritate the skin.

An alternative is to soak your nail in your first morning urine. When you first get up, capture your urine in a bowl. Put your finger or toes in the urine for 10 minutes each day, for up to 3 weeks. This will speed the healing, and it will actually work on its own. (Many cultures use urine therapy for a wide range of ills such as pink eye, abrasions, and burns. The first urine is the most acidic, and it is from your body so it won't hurt you.)

---

6 An herbal formula is a mixture of herbs for a specific purpose.

This type of fungus can spread to other toes or fingernails, so it is important to treat it immediately. Since it is hard to get rid of, be patient, as a cure may be weeks or months away.

Tip 6 - Antiperspirants or Deodorants

Avoid the use of antiperspirants. Not only do they contain aluminum and other harmful chemicals, they also block the flow of toxins out of the body, redirecting them to the breast area. Imagine the lymph draining down toward the underarms and the breasts; when the underarm is blocked, the toxins can't leave the body, so the lymphatic system can't complete its job. The increase in breast cancers in both men and women could have a relation to this blockage along with tight bras and other clothing. (Don't forget to move the lymph with exercise as well; unlike the heart, the lymph doesn't have a pump to move it along. When you are sedentary, so is the lymph. Jump on a mini-trampoline.)

You can find natural deodorants made from herbs which are wonderfully effective. Look at the same local stores and websites that you have explored for

Have you heard of deodorant crystals? These crystals work very well and an added bonus is that they last for years.

A friend of mine visited India recently and was amazed to find that the women with no running water traveled to the Ganges River (very polluted) to gather a bowl of water. They swiped a crystal (the same type as the deodorant stones) through the water two or three times, and the contaminants fell to the bottom of the bowl, making clear water for drinking! So, when you take a bath in chlorinated, fluoridated city or community water, run your deodorant stone through it for safety. Some companies such as Global Light sell a stir wand that they say 'maximizes your water's hydration potential.'

Natural Recipes for Face and Skin Care

"Beauty is as Beauty Does."

Making your own skin care products with natural ingredients such as avocado, lemons and oranges, milk and honey, beeswax, and organic oils is much easier than you might think. Below are some very simple recipes[7] for you to try out on yourself; it won't take long for you to discover the wonderful relief the body experiences when we no longer slather on chemical-laden soaps, shampoos, and lotions.

In all cases, the best way to clean the face is with a cheap washcloth from Wal Mart; these white wash cloths are the economy brand and are found in packs of 6 or 10. Scrub the face (not too vigorously) to exfoliate – no need for anything else!

These facial treatments are for skin tightening and closing pores:

Green Clay Face Mask

1/4 c. green clay powder 1 t. raw honey
Enough water to make a smooth paste. Apply to skin and allow to dry completely before rinsing. Remove with a wash cloth and warm water.

Egg White Face Mask

Separate egg yolk from white. Whip the whites with a fork for 1 minute. Apply to face and allow to dry completely. Remove with a wash cloth and warm water for tighter, firmer skin.

These facial treatments are moisturizing:

Oatmeal Face Mask

Cook 1/2 cup oatmeal. You may want to mash or blend. Cool. Add 1/4 cup raw honey and mix thoroughly.

---

[7] Some of the recipes came, in part, from the book by Mike Hurburt and Anna Carter, *Pure Beauty.*

Spread on face and neck and leave on for 20-30 minutes.

Avocado Face Mask

Mash 1 ripe avocado.

Add 1/2 t. honey

1/2 t. lemon juice

5 drops sandalwood or orange essential oil.

Apply to face for a soothing, moisture mask. Leave on 20 minutes and rinse.

Fruit and Veggie Facial

Clean your face with warm water; take off make up with almond oil or coconut oil.

Use organic apple cider vinegar as an astringent and to moisturize the hands and face.

Grind sunflower, sesame, and pumpkin seeds in a blender until

rough for facial scrub.

White or green clay powder can be mixed with water to make a paste; apply a thin layer to skin and allow to dry completely. You may powder oatmeal or calendula flowers and add to clay mixture. Cucumber slices really do soothe the eyes and the skin surrounding them, so while your mask is hardening, put cucumber slices over the eyes and take a lie down for 20 minutes. Then rinse with warm water.

Mash or blend avocado (add raw honey if you like) and put on the face as a moisture mask. Leave on 20 minutes.

Other Ideas

Make a finishing mask with lightly whipped egg white; allow to dry completely to close pores. Rinse with warm water.

Slice an organic beet – color lips and cheeks with this.

Use only organic lip gloss and color.

Tooth Powder

3 T. green clay powder, 1 T. baking soda

5 drops tea tree oil

1 drop peppermint or wintergreen oil 1 T. sea salt

Mix ingredients in a blender or with a mortar and pestle. Store in a glass container for up to one week.

Mouthwash

1/2 c. food-grade peroxide

1/2 c. vodka or Everclear

1 1/2 c. distilled water

10 drops tea tree oil

2 drops peppermint or wintergreen

Use morning and evening to keep mouth free of harmful bacteria and to clear up any gum or tooth issues. For persistent problems, use Essential Herb Tooth and Gum Tonic.

Sweet Basil Mouth Wash

Pick 2 cups fresh basil.

Pour vodka to cover and use a tight lid.

Store in a dark cabinet or out of direct light.

Every day, turn bottle over several times, for three weeks.

At the end of the three weeks, strain the liquid into a separate jar; add 2 cups distilled water and 1/2 c. food- grade hydrogen peroxide. Use as a mouthwash; if you would like it more dilute, add more water. Store in a cool place.

Bath Oil

1 c. sweet almond oil

1/2 c. glycerin (optional)

1/2 c. liquid castile soap

1 essential oil blend (see below)

Mix and pour 1/4 c. of bath oil under running bath water.

This oil doesn't float on the top; it disappears into the water and is absorbed by the skin. Here are some essential oil blends for you to consider:

Want a Relaxing blend?

Try one of these: 20 drops chamomile, 15 drops sandalwood, 15 drops cedar wood, 15 drops lavender, or 10 drops lemongrass.

Want a Stimulating blend?

Try one of these: 20 drops rosemary, 15 drops patchouli, 15 drops spearmint or wintergreen, 6 drops ginger, 15 drops spearmint, or 15 drops rosemary.

Hair Rinses

4 chamomile tea bags or 4 T. chamomile

2 c. distilled water

1/4 c. fresh rosemary

2 T. apple cider vinegar

Bring the water to boil in a saucepan.

Pour over fresh rosemary and chamomile.

Cover and let steep for at least 15 minutes.

Add the vinegar; strain off the herbs.

After shampooing hair, pour over head to remove build-up of shampoos and products.

Leave on 2-3 minutes.

Rinse with warm water.

Scar Essential Oil Formula
10 drops Helichrysum
6 drops Lavender
8 drops Lemongrass
4 drops Patchouli
5 drops Myrrh
1 oz. carrier oil/ jojoba oil

Next Steps

Here are your Next Steps to support your body:

☐ Go through your skin care, make up, hair products and deodorants. Check the labels for preservatives such as alcohols, or colors with numbers and any chemicals you don't recognize. Put them all in a basket to throw away, put in the guest bathroom, or donate to a Shelter.

☐ Start looking for substitutes based upon natural ingredients. You will love the new more natural you! Find your local health food store and support a local business, or go online for brands such as Dessert Essence, Boom, NOW, or begin to experiment with making your own?

☐ Buy a bristle brush and some liquid coconut oil. Start to brush each day.

☐ Buy two or three essential oils locally or visit Mountain Rose Herbs, Doterra or Young Living Oils on the internet. For example, Rosemary (invigorating), Lavender (calming), and Peppermint (stimulating)

☐ Buy these key ingredients and follow some of the recipes:

  o Baking Soda, Organic, EV Coconut Oil

  o Castille Soaps and natural clays

☐ Research these products and add them to your budget or gift list:

  o A filter on your shower head to remove chlorine, fluoride and other harmful chemicals.

  o A Neti pot

  o A tongue scraper

☐ Your skin is alive and needs to be fed with healthy oils and healthy diet.

Week Two: Take Steps to Balance your pH

Your body is constantly adjusting to your diet and your life-style. Your blood must maintain a pH of 7.3 to 7.4 so if you are eating and living an acid lifestyle then your body pulls alkaline substances (e.g. calcium) from the bones, teeth, and tissues which causes issues over time.

pH is a measure of acidity. The pH scale measures **how acidic or basic** a substance is. It ranges from 0 to 14. A pH of 7 is neutral. A high number is alkaline. A low number is acidic. For example, diet soda is often 2.5 pH; we have all heard the stories of using diet soda as an acidic cleaning fluid.

Modern diets feature packaged and processed foods, sugars and refined carbohydrates, flesh foods (beef, pork, fish), and caffeine. These are all acidic (low pH) and put pressure on the body to maintain the correct pH in the blood.

In addition, viruses, bacteria and fungi thrive in a low or acidic pH. Cancer has been associated with low pH (acidic), and there are many claims that cancer cells cannot survive in a balanced pH alkaline environment.

And when the pH is out of range, the body cannot absorb key minerals. Chronic diseases result when a person's body is depleted of electrolytes: sodium, magnesium, potassium and calcium – the body's natural buffering minerals. Do you have any of these complaints?

Weight gain or low energy
Kidney and bladder infections
Immune system issues
Heart and lung weakness
Aging, lifeless skin and hair
Weak bones (the blood steals calcium from the bones)
Joint pain, inflammation, arthritis, fibroids, gout
Fibromyalgia

These depleting conditions come on gradually and may be affecting a person for many years before they manifest, usually as a dramatic and painful set of symptoms.

Just think for a minute about vegetable gardens. Every gardener knows that the balance of acid and alkaline in any organism is of extreme importance. If tomatoes yellow and collect aphids, the gardener knows that the soil isn't properly balanced. Instead of letting the plants shrivel up and die or spraying them with poisons for a temporary fix, the smart gardener knows to add organic compost (balanced food) for nourishment and crab meal, bone meal, or lime for alkalinity – to raise the pH. Within a short while, most plants are blooming and producing healthy food.

It seems a no brainer to me that we could learn a lot from our plants. Shouldn't we be adding nutritious foods to alkalize and energize the human body as well?

Dr. Robert Young in his book *The pH Miracle* uses the image of an aquarium to explain the importance of balance in nature; with a more neutral pH, the water is crystal clear, but when it becomes off balance, murky green slime begins to grow along the sides. Just imagine that this is your body and that you too are an aquarium with glass sides; after all we are 70% water! Would your insides be crystal clear, or would they be a bit murky? Are you in need of some nutritional changes to bring you back to clarity?

Many believe that to maintain good health we need a state of alkalinity in our tissues; and we can achieve this by choosing foods and a lifestyle that help to adjust the relative pH of the body.

Your Goals

Here is a summary of the best ways for you make your body more alkaline. We will get into the details in the next Chapters. Your goal is to make all of these changes eventually. Do you do any of these already?

- ☐ Drink restructured, ionized, alkaline water if it is available to you. If not, invest in a good filter. Do not carry or drink water in plastic bottles!

- ☐ Invest in a water ionizer/filter and bottle your own water in stainless, glass, or heavy, BPA-free plastic or add alkaline drops to filtered water.

- ☐ At least, install a filter under your sink or invest in a Berky water filter for clean, filtered and safer water.

- ☐ Make your long-term goal a diet that is 80-85% alkaline and eat the alkaline foods from the charts.

- ☐ Decide where the acids are most affecting you and what your weakest link is: sinus, lungs, gut, or joints.

- ☐ Drink 1/2 lemon with cayenne pepper in 16 oz. of warm water every morning, warm or room temperature.

- ☐ Drink carrots, celery, beets and greens diluted half-and-half with water, blended into a smoothie.

- ☐ Soak 20 - 30 minutes in a bath containing 1 cup Epsom salts one day and 1 box baking soda and/or ginger tea or powder the next.

- ☐ Exercise.

- ☐ Take cold showers, laugh a lot, and love many.

- ☐ Continue with your conversion to a more natural lifestyle by brushing your skin, using only natural skin, teeth, and hair care products.

Tip 1 – Avoid Eating Chemicals in Fake Food

"Whatever Miss T. eats, Turns into Miss T" – Walter de la Mare

Pay attention to how often you are being sold 'fake food' and watch how you consume acid-producing processed foods such as white flour and sugar, coffee, tea and soft drinks.

Artificial chemical sweeteners like NutraSweet, Splenda, Equal, or aspartame are some of the most acid-forming "foods" available. If you have a "sweet tooth," then you would be better to use organic honey, Grade B Maple Syrup or Stevia, an herb that is used as a sweetener.

Artificial creamers are acid forming. If you want dairy in your coffee and tea, then drink organic almond, coconut, or whole-fat milk, unless you are lactose intolerant. Eat organic butter, not artificial margarine and fake butter substitutes.

Foods labeled 'Low Fat' are full of sugar and salt to add back the lost flavor, and these highly processed foods are acid-forming chemicals in your body.

Avoid sliced meats, sausages and bacon that are high in nitrates, a chemical that preserves the meat but think what it does inside your body! Shop for nitrate free meats, now more available in regular stores.

Once you start to pay attention, you will realize that the supermarket is full of aisles of highly- processed, fake "food" and fake "drinks." Next time you shop, walk around the outside of the store to find fruit, vegetables, and real meats. In the center of the store, you will find aisle after aisle of Franken-foods. Eat things that grew that way naturally. A carrot grew that way; a bag of chips did not.

Give yourself permission to eat organic real food, and avoid the low-fat lie!

Obesity is the normal bodily response to over- acidification. Fat cells bind to acids and carry them away from the vital organs to protect them from the degrading effects of acid. In a slightly alkaline environment, the body will reach an ideal weight and better health.

Tip 2 – Load up on Vegetables

Here's the bottom line, vegetables and fruits are more alkaline than meats and chemicals. Generally speaking, load up your plate with 80% fresh organic vegetables and alkaline fruits, and eat 20% of the high-protein more acidic foods. You can eat what you want, just keep it in proportion.

For example, think about a typical plate in a restaurant with 6oz of meat, a side of broccoli, and a small house salad. Imagine picking up the meat in one hand and the vegetables in the other hand and comparing their weight? Think about how many more vegetables you would have to eat, for them to weigh four times heavier than the meat! The solution? Just cut the meat; enjoy the smaller piece and take the rest home.

Meats are all acidifying, which has been long understood, yet many fad diets today encourage us to eat no grain and much more protein. They want us to avoid the sugar and starch while loading us up with acidifying proteins. I have always heard that gout is the "rich man's disease" because only the rich could afford meats. In recent years, Dr. Colin Campbell writes in *The China Study* about his experiences serving the NIH with the "rich" families in the Philippines. He discovered that only the wealthier children were getting cancer. The main differences, you guessed it, meat consumption! Acidic foods aren't necessarily bad foods, but if you eat 80% off of the acid side of the chart, you just might need to rethink your diet and your health. Processed foods, sweets, meats, and refined carbohydrates tend to be acid, while fresh fruits and vegetables result in alkalinity. Better yet, change what you like and enjoy the better health that comes along with the "alkalarian way" of life.

In a later chapter, we will list acid and alkaline foods: remember, eat real food, mostly plants, and you'll be just fine.

Tip 3 - Test Your Own pH!

You can take control of your own health by testing your own pH at home, and see how your body reacts as you make changes to your water, food, and lifestyle.

How do you do this? First, you need to buy some pHydrion paper or "pH strips". Just look online for pH strips. This is a narrow strip of paper that changes color when it is wet, and the color indicates the degree of acidity or alkalinity in the urine and saliva. You want to buy narrow range (5-8) pH strips that come with a color chart that lets you identify the pH reading; yellow is acidic and deep blue is alkaline. (Available at http://takestepstohealth.com)

First thing upon waking, test your saliva by spitting on the pH paper. Note the color change, compare to the color guide on the container, and write down the pH number. Do this before brushing your teeth, drinking, smoking, or even thinking of eating any food. The optimum saliva pH should be 6.4 to stay healthy and prevent disease.

Next, test your first urine of the morning. This is urine that has been stored in your bladder during the night that is ready to be eliminated when you get up. You need to urinate on a strip of pH paper, note the color change and compare it to the color chart, and write down the pH number for your records. The first urine should be 6.4 or a bit lower.

Is your first urine pH lower than 6.4? Your first urine is acidic; a slightly acidic reading is normal for the first morning urine, as your body is throwing off acids from the day before instead of storing them. However, you might be deficient in alkaline buffers and need to consume alkaline ionized water and move to a more alkaline diet rich in fresh green vegetables and fruits.

Is your first urine pH higher than 6.4? Your first urine is alkaline. Your body may not be repairing itself overnight and is trying to neutralize the acids produced by physical, mental and emotional stress and from metabolic processes from the day before.

To balance the pH of the urine, you need to move away from acidic foods and drinks and begin ingesting liberal amounts of alkaline ionized water and electron-rich green vegetables, low sugar fruits, healthy fats and balanced calciums. Most people who purchase or even sell calcium supplements are unaware that different calciums have different effects in the body; calcium carbonate is alkalizing but calcium lactate is acidifying, for example. Calcium from dark leafy greens would have an assortment (balanced), whereas a supplement from rocks might be just one type.

When you can, test your second morning urine before eating any food. The acids should be gone the second time you urinate, so your urine pH should be ideally about 6.4 – 6.5. If the pH is lower than 6.4, then you are in a state of latent tissue acidosis, and you are deficient in alkaline buffers such as bicarbonate, sodium, potassium, and magnesium. The lower pH is also indicative of a diet high in animal protein and refined carbohydrates and thus an increase in the level of acids produced from metabolizing these foods. These acids include nitric, sulfuric, phosphoric, and uric acids.

To build your alkaline reserves, consume at least ½ oz. per day of alkaline ionized water per pound of body weight, and/or drink fresh lemon water and eliminate or reduce high protein (high acid) from dairy, beef, chicken, turkey, pork and fish to normalize your pH.

Another way to test your alkalizing buffer system is to eat a raw almond after testing your first saliva of the day. Chew the raw almond up well and wait 5 minutes to repeat the saliva test. This time the saliva should test approximately 8 to 8.5 on the test strips because the body has released stored buffers into the saliva to buffer the acids in the almond, which is slightly acidic. If you do not see the test strips turn dark blue (8 to 8.5 pH), then this is an indication that you are low in minerals and other acid buffers and need to make changes in your lifestyle.

Eating an 80% alkaline food diet and reducing stress should help your body correct any imbalance.

What is the Importance of this pH Testing?

How well you treat yourself in general determines how effectively the salivary glands, pancreas, gallbladder and liver will be able to handle excess acidity. So, testing your pH will directly show you the results of your taking steps to improve your health.

In the morning, the pH of your urine and saliva will show the overall state of your health and the condition of the alkaline reserves of your body, which reflects the diet you have been eating and the fluids you have been consuming over the last days, weeks, months, and years. This pH number stays rather constant and will only change after some time and effort has been spent in alkalizing and energizing the body. The efficiency of the digestive system in dealing with what you ate the night before is shown by morning readings. When you begin to alkalize, you will see the morning pH of the urine and saliva become pH of 6.8 to 7.2, but unless you are eating vegan with a lot of dark green vegetables, you'll see pH level at about 6.4-6.6.

After one eats, the stomach releases the necessary HCL (acid) to help digest the food. The pancreas secretes an equivalent amount of base or sodium bicarbonate (alkaline – 11.5) that is picked up by the blood stream and delivered to the alkaline glands of the body: the saliva, the pancreas, the gallbladder, the pylorus glands in the duodenum and the liver. The maximum amount of base (alkaline) in the blood and therefore in the urine and saliva occurs one to two hours after you eat. Therefore, in the evening, the pH of your urine and saliva will reflect your lifestyle for that particular day.

Overnight, your body should be working to flush out all the acids generated in a day of digestion, respiration, metabolism and degeneration, and that will be reflected in the pH of your morning saliva and urine.

If these acids are not all flushed out during the night, they accumulate, day after day. Over time, the body (blood) will desperately try to maintain the alkaline fluid pH (blood) at 7.365 by eliminating acids through the bowels, urinary system, lungs and skin. If not, the acids settle in the weakest parts of the body and are bound to fat and stored on our fingers, knees, hips, thighs, stomach, breasts and brain. Bottom-line... most symptomologies are the result of excess acids retained in the body, which is ultimately the direct cause of ALL sickness and ALL disease.

But if you measure the pH of your saliva and urine, then you can immediately see the effects on your body of your choices on how to live, eat and drink, and how it determines the quality and quantity of your life. You should monitor your saliva and urine each day for at least 12 weeks or until you establish your balanced pH at 6.4-6.6.

Complete the pH Record Chart

Create a chart like this to keep track of the pH of your urine and saliva for 12 weeks. (Or download a chart from TakeStepsToHealth.com). Pay attention in the notes to how the pH readings reflect your lifestyle choices.

	Morning		Evening		
Date	Urine pH	Saliva pH	Urine pH	Saliva PH	Notes (diet, stress)

Remember that Hyper-acidity equals Dis-ease. An acid body experiences rashes, headaches, diarrhea and constipation, which later develop into heart, thyroid, liver or joint problems. If we stay acidic and the cells are deprived of oxygen, we can become very sick. The body has to work to rid itself of trash from the breaking down of food before it can work to rid itself of trouble of any kind. So, plan your meals based on the 80% alkaline and 20% acid rule. The less junk in the body, the easier it is for the blood to stay alkaline.

Take Steps to Eat The Balanced pH Way

"It's not what you do, it's what you do every day"- Betty Sue O'Brian

It doesn't matter "what you do" occasionally so, yes, you can eat that piece of birthday cake. It matters what you do every day; do you eat cake every day? Try to follow the 80:20 rule every day and your health will improve.

Here is a list of which foods are alkaline and which foods are acid. Take the list to the grocery store and purchase plenty of items on the alkaline side of the chart. Don't forget that organic is better; standards are in place to help us be certain the certified organic is really organic. Basically, green foods, most plant foods, many fruits and some seeds, nuts and oils are alkaline. Flesh foods, dairy and synthetic ingredients such as artificial sweeteners and hydrogenated fats are acidic.

Your 80:20 Food Guide[8]

Don't deprive yourself but do pay attention to what you eat, and give your body a balanced diet. Plan to eat 80% of your daily food from the left-hand Alkaline column and 20% of your daily intake from the right-hand Acidic column. Since most of the alkaline based foods are fruits and vegetables, which promote health and weight loss, people who try to follow this general rule find they have more energy and seek their ideal weight without "dieting." I like to call it the *Alkaline Live-it!* In addition, you will find many charts out there with conflicting information. Remember it is how the food is burned in the process of digestion. Some charts measure the pH of the food itself. Don't worry too much about it...if

---

[8] Chart largely from the work of Dr. Robert Young. Emoto, Masaru. *The True Power of Water. Healing and Discovering Ourselves.* New York: Atria Books, 2003.

the food is a vegetable, eat it. Eat real food, mostly vegetables. It is not necessary to eliminate foods other than highly processed, plastic foods!

Eat 80% of these 'Alkaline' foods		Eat 20% of these 'Acidic' foods	
Fresh lemon	Fresh Lime	Cantaloupe	Tangerines
Cherries	Umeboshi plum	Dates	Mango
Coconut, fresh	Carrots	Plums	Papaya
Watermelon	Grapefruit	Raspberries	Apricot
Fresh bananas		Blueberries	Peach
Sour apples		Strawberries	Pear
		Cranberries	Banana, ripe
		Grapes	Pineapple, ripe
Soy beans		White & Brown Rice	
Navy and		Wheat	
Lima beans		Wheat Bread	
Miso		White Bread	
Buckwheat		Whole Grain Bread	
Lentils		Rye Bread	
Millet and quinoa			
Almonds		Pistachios	Cashews
Sesame seeds		Peanuts	Walnuts
Bee Pollen - Royal Jelly		Fresh Water Fish	Eggs
Spirulina (blue/green algae).		Ocean Fish	Liver
		Oysters	Chicken
Chlorella (algae)/spirulina		Hard Cheese	Beef
Cesium: pH 14		Cottage Cheese	Pork
Potassium: pH 14		Feta Cheese	Turkey
		Homogenized Milk	
Sodium: pH 14		Buttermilk Butter	
Calcium: pH 7 - 12		Yogurt	
Magnesium: pH 9		Avoid fake creamer	
Fish oils		Margarine	
Olive oil		Corn Oil	
Coconut Oil		Vegetable Oils	
Avocado oil		Avoid Canola Oil	
Sesame oil		Ketchup	
Cayenne peppers		Vinegar	
Vegetable Juices		Soy sauce	
Ginger		Mustard	
Horseradish		Mayonnaise	

Eat 80% of these 'Alkaline' foods	Eat 20% of these 'Acidic' foods
Organic raw honey Raw Stevia	Brown rice syrup Sugar Fructose or Turbinado Sugar cane (Sucanat) Molasses Beet sugar White sugar Chocolate (pick dark chocolate) Avoid Artificial sweeteners
Alkaline water Green tea Herbal teas Lemon water	Black Tea Hard Liquor Beer Wine Coffee (except for fresh-brewed which might be an antioxidant)
Eat mostly (organic) vegetables. These are the most alkaline: Alfalfa, & Radish sprouts Arugula Asparagus Avocado Barley Grass Beets Bell Peppers Broccoli Brussels Sprouts Buckwheat Cabbage Carrots Cauliflower Cayenne peppers Celery Celery Cherries Chives Coconut, fresh Collard Greens Dandelion leaves Eggplant Endive Green Beans	Green Beans Horseradish Kelp Kohlrabi Leeks Lettuce Okra Onion Parsnips Pumpkin Radishes Red Cabbage Rutabaga Soy Beans Spinach Squash Tomato Peas Turnip Greens Turnips Vegetable Juices Watercress Watermelon Wheat grass Zucchini (Frozen, canned, and processed foods are more acidic.)

Were you surprised to see lemons and limes in the Alkaline column? Yes, they are acidic, but they have an alkaline reaction inside your digestive system. In the next chapter, we will learn more about the benefits of adding lemon and limes to your diet.

Tip – Be Open to Change

Many people, when advised to follow an alkaline eating plan, read the instructions and come back the next week saying something such as, "What else have you got to offer me? I can't do this because my meals are all planned around meat and potatoes." Or, "This won't work for us because we eat out three to five nights a week." Not too many readily follow the 80/20 (80% alkaline and 20% acid) rule. But if a person's very life is threatened, or he or she is overtaken with yeast, viruses and the accompanying misery, the situation often changes because now ANYTHING would be better than exhaustion or certain death. This causes people to reflect on whether they are at all serious about their health, longevity, or quality of life if they have to have the threat of death before taking sensible eating seriously. Again, a person may have to change what he or she likes.

High acidity can affect all body systems; pH balance maintains alkaline reserves that are used to meet energy demands. There is so much more acid waste because of the SAD diet that our bodies can't handle it all. We are now fat, not only because of overeating, but also because of our body's responses to having to handle so much acid waste. My state, Mississippi, is now the fattest in the nation because many eat fried chicken and potato salad and drink sweet tea ... with a high acid pH.

If your urinary pH stays between 6.2-6.4 in the morning and 6.8 and 7 in the evening, your body is functioning within a normal range. Yet many people who begin an alkalizing program find their pH at 6 or below which is a range where illness occurs. Certainly, people can get the pH too alkaline as well, but those who eat the SAD diet will probably not have this problem. If you find your urine and saliva are staying above 7, you might need to add some apple cider vinegar with meals to help balance your pH.

Tip – Drink Alkaline Water

One of the best things people can do to correct over acidity is to clean up the diet and lifestyle and drink alkaline water. Humans are about 70% water, so the fluids we put in our body might be even more important than we ever thought possible.

Loading up on bottled water with an acid pH and poisons from plastics is self-defeating – isn't it a shame that so many Americans are trying to do the right thing by drinking water, yet the plastic bottles and the acidified water in them create another set of health issues. Check the pH of the commercial bottled water sold at over $1.00 for a 16-oz. bottle; it is usually just about as acidic as Sprite and all of the "nutritious" sports drinks. Around the world people are realizing that plastic water bottles are a source of environmental pollution; now we know they might pollute the human body as well. Read the bottles: you might be surprised to find that the water came from a municipal water system (such as your own tap water). Tap water is probably not the answer. When Dr. Emoto studied the crystalline shapes of tap water, he found very few that were well formed, meaning that they wouldn't provide the body the hydration it needs. In his books, *The Hidden Messages in Water* and *The True Power of Water*, he illustrates how important our water is and explains that it can actually be "imprinted" with messages such as "I love you," or "I hate you" to change the quality of the contents.[9]

---

[9] Emoto, Masaru. *The True Power of Water. Healing and Discovering Ourselves.* New York: Atria Books, 2003.

Over acidification of the blood indirectly causes dis-ease. An acid terrain creates weakened cells and affects our nervous system (anxiety and depression), our muscles (lack of tone and atrophy), our skin tone (wrinkles and age spots), our brain (forgetfulness and lack of clarity), and our organs (weak). Most often, people who are suffering from illness have a low pH; Dr. Robert Young, in one of his newsletters, even goes so far as to say that most winter "flu" is really just hyper-acidity from holiday dining on sugars and low-quality foods. Not "catching" the flu would be reason enough to consider eating more alkalizing foods.

Follow These Dietary Guidelines:

- ☐ The lighter the better – fruit and vegetable smoothies in the morning (See *Going Green...the Smoothie Way* for serious health-increasing recipes).

- ☐ Good clean water and no liquids during or right after meals; stay hydrated!

- ☐ Eat meals during digestive friendly times: 12 until 7 p.m.

- ☐ Combine good properly:

    - o Veggies and animal protein – good together.
    - o Veggies and starch – good
    - o Starch and animal protein – <u>not</u> good together.

- ☐ Eat all fruits alone except in smoothies made in a Vita Mix or 3 horsepower blender.

- ☐ Buy organic! Free range and raw.

- ☐ Get sunshine on the head for at least 15 minutes a day to enliven the mood, restore the pineal gland, and to help manufacture Vitamin D.

* If you feel confused about pH, it is because there is a lot of conflicting information out there and the jury is still out on exactly how it works. The body MAINTAINS pH to keep you healthy; we can best help the body by eating a plant-based diet and avoiding an overabundance of acidifying foods. Enough said.

Next Steps

Here are your Next Steps to balance your pH:

☐ Check the label on your bottled water and consider getting an alkaline, ionizing water device such as Kangen water or a water restructuring device such as Utopic or Ultimate water. It may be the single most important investment you can make. Otherwise, get a charcoal filter and bottle your water in a metal or glass container to carry with you, and buy alkalizing drops for your drinking water.

☐ Write messages of love and gratitude on the bottle to improve the vibration of the water you drink. Don't drink out of recyclable plastic bottles. Check out My Sigg or Klean Kanteen for a nice drinking bottle, or use glass bottles.

☐ Get your body pH balanced ASAP. Clear up your "fish tank" by choosing alkaline foods and drinking alkaline, not acid, water. Maintain a healthy pH and limit the amount of flesh foods (acidic) and refined carbs (acidic) that you eat.

☐ EAT RAW. The percentage of raw foods in your diet correlates strongly with your overall health picture.

☐ Essential: EXERCISE every day.

☐ Feed the brain and pituitary with sunlight for 15 minutes per day.

☐ Light up your body with natural, energizing light from the sun.

☐ And if you really want to understand the importance of pH and energy, pay a visit to Dr. Jerry Tennant's website: www.tennantinstitute.com to learn about cleaning up your body so that you won't host undesirable bugs and virus.

Week Three: Our Food Supply – How Safe is it?

Your Goals

☐ Eat more raw salads, fruits and vegetables and make more raw smoothies.

☐ Eat living foods and consider converting to ancient, alkaline grains, preferably non-hybridized.

☐ Eat more vegetables and fruits; transition to a healthy diet over time to feel your best throughout the process

☐ Eat organic; demand it.

☐ Make conscious changes to glass and stainless steel cookware instead of plastic, Teflon, and aluminum.

Flesh Eaters

☐ Are you eating too much meat (acidic)?

☐ Are you eating it from the wrong source (meat that has been treated with chemicals and hormones, or artificially fatted)

☐ Consider cruelty to food lot animals – is their consciousness and fear in the food you choose?

☐ Fats dissolve fats; like dissolves like is a rule in chemistry. Are you getting enough of the right kind of fats in your diet each day?

Our Food Supply – How Safe Is It?

"Love God with all your heart and love your neighbor as yourself" - Jesus

Why is it important to change our diets? You might say, "I'm eating more vegetables and fruits, and I eat salmon two times a week. I never eat beef, and I have substituted soy milk for cow's milk. Isn't that enough?

Well, herein lies the problem. Are the vegetables organic or at least cleaned as much as possible? Is the salmon wild Alaskan or farm-raised Atlantic (not wild but grain fed)? Have you investigated processed soy and its damaging effects on the thyroid gland? Oh, and if you are eating more chicken, one of the most mucus-producing foods available, is it making you feel good, or are your allergies and arthritis "acting up" a bit?

More than at any time before, Americans are trying to eat right and get fit, but much confusion surrounds just what is healthy. When people really care about their health and try to uncover the best practices, the amount of information out there is overwhelming at times. Eating a balanced diet may not be good enough in today's climate of big agribusiness and big-pharma. Maybe we wish to be completely healthy while still eating hydrogenated fat (in almost all processed foods), eating tons of sugar (nine teaspoons in a Coke), while drinking alcohol and coffee, bread and chips. Just today I looked at every cookie in the grocery store trying to find ONE without hydrogenated fats or partially hydrogenated fats. Results? Not one. Maybe we could do enough exercise, drink enough water, and do enough yoga... or maybe not.

The good news is that it is possible to be healthy almost regardless of what we eat. Just get lined up with Godliness and cleanliness of thought, word and deed, and whatever we eat will carry our health a long way. Live on the energy of God. Be a Breatharian. Don't take unnecessary drugs, prescription or otherwise, drink plenty of clean, alkaline water. Voila! You are a healthy person. When we are in the "zone" and truly connected with Spirit, we might be able to get away with not eating so carefully. I have been amazed to see some elderly folks in good health who don't watch their diet much. Usually, these are people who are moderate, volunteer to help others, and love unconditionally – oh, and born many years ago, they lived before the world became so completely synthetic and quite possibly had a healthier start in life. Studies done on volunteerism showed that those who help others live longer, happier lives. And, happy people don't get sick much; if you don't believe it, take a look at people who are falling in love. They stay as healthy as can be!

God sends signals that support the entire universe – when we are at-one-ment with God, we can be comfortable in our bodies, but when we get out of alignment with Spirit, we might experience dis-ease or dis-comfort. Jesus told us to love God with all our heart and love our neighbor as ourselves; this is the greatest commandment. Of course, this doesn't mean that if we are sick, we are "sinful" or doing something wrong, but as it says in the Bible, "A happy heart is good medicine."

I cannot discuss this topic without telling you about my mother, one beautiful woman who has inspired my life. Momma was an angel on earth to me. She had been born the weaker identical twin and suffered from many childhood illnesses such as rheumatic fever and later polio. While lying in her bed as a child, she vowed to devote her life to helping others if she survived. She became a nurse, and when my father abandoned us, she raised four children by herself, working night shifts and double shifts to keep food on the table. This didn't stop her from attending PTA meetings at school or sports events when she could. When my father came back after being away for almost twenty years, Momma raised his daughter, my sister Lynda, as her own. She just did not distinguish ownership or pass judgment, and even when we barely had food on the table, she always made room at the table for anyone we brought home. Several times, she took people into our home that needed a place to live for a while. We now joke about the fact that she smoked cigarettes until she was eighty, and told everyone how easy it was to quit, to just lay the cigarettes down and think about something else. She ate a lot of Snickers and marshmallow peanuts, but tiny meals. Oh, and she drank coffee, too. As a side note, we rarely ate meat. She gave us vitamins and other supplements back in the 60's. The point is that there seems to be a connection between goodness, kindness, love and happiness that transcends biology and heredity. When we tackle our health, we have to incorporate the whole being: as Caroline Myass says, "Our biography becomes our biology."

Now, assuming that most people are not at-one–ment with God or totally satisfied with their lives, jobs, and their health, discovering what health habits will most help them stay strong into old age certainly becomes more important. Remember, the SAD surely is not the answer. The next time you are around an elderly man or woman who is shrinking with age, notice how much milk and other dairy he or she is drinking, supposedly for better bones! There seems to be an inverse ratio: the more milk they drink, the more they shrink up. Cow's milk is much better for baby cows.

Randall Fitzgerald's book, *The Hundred Year Lie*[10], outlines the stages of the "Slippery Slope Index" from 1900 – 1998, demonstrating how synthetics in manufacturing have ruined our food supply. In the 40's everyone loved convenience foods – margarine that never spoiled and solid peanut butter, but by 1998, the long-range health effects were more than apparent. Fast forward to 2017 when Americans are ignorantly eating GMO foods that have been sprayed at harvest with glycophates (Round Up). Watch *What the Wheat* on Netflix.

Fitzgerald refers to the adage "Better life through chemistry" used at Disney in the Monsanto exhibit in the 60's. As early as 1900, chemists were

---

[10] Fitzgerald, Randal. *The Hundred Year Lie. How Food and Medicine are Destroying Your Life.* New York: Penguin, 2006.

creating artificial sugars and butter replacements, adding MSG and creating hydrogenated fats for vegetable shortening and margarine. This was a retailer's greatest joy; indefinite shelf life. Even today, "Monsanto, the $10 billion corporation at the forefront of GE research, has also created 'Round-up Ready' seeds to allow ever-increasing applications of this herbicide...."[11] I asked a Doctor who was "farming" in the Mississippi Delta about his crop and whether he had considered organic farming. "Heck no," he said. "I use the Round Up impregnated seeds." Now try to wash that off of your bell pepper!

Synthetics changed our lives: synthetic clothes, food wrap, preservatives, supplements, bottles, and medications. However, with these changes that have made life easier, has come an increase in many degenerative diseases and cancers. As Fitzgerald claims, "The cure is NOT more chemicals." Instead he suggests that we buy organic produce and shop the stores that are making the effort to provide safe, organic, non-GMO fruits and vegetables. Support smaller companies that are making the effort to turn this situation around. Statistics abound concerning the effect that our poisonous environment has had on our health.[12] Now we are bombarded with formaldehyde, polyurethane, and other chemicals in the fiber of our walls, floors and carpeting; these have contributed to the huge increase in xenoestrogens which mimic estrogens and are suspected to cause breast lumps, prostate enlargement, cysts and polyps, early puberty, and other health issues.

In 1900, cancer was the leading cause of deaths, but now it is the cause of 1 in 5 deaths; that number has doubled, and the same doubling has occurred with diabetes. From 1920 on, the production of synthetic chemicals increased from under one million pounds a year to 140 billion pounds each year. In 1930, 3,000

---

[11] Fitzgerald, Randal. *The Hundred Year Lie. How Food and Medicine are Destroying Your Life.* New York: Penguin, 2006.

[12] Sadeki, Mark. "Better Living Through Chemistry." Sermonette on February 23, 2008. The First Universalist Society in Franklin's Green Committee Blog. Fusfgreen.typepad.com. Accessed February 23, 2008.

people died of heart disease, and today the number is over 700,000. Another interesting statistic involves the decrease in sperm counts in humans. From 1938 until 1990 sperm counts dropped by 50%. Could chemicals in food, water and air be to blame?[13]

Naturally occurring health is not only possible, it is our birth right. Radical regeneration is also possible, no doubt about that! But you will have to come to terms with the impact of the synthetics belief system on your life and the lives of all those you love. Each of us has to begin to research "green building" and organic fabrics. In the next chapter, cleaning up your cleaning products will help to lessen the number of these foreign chemicals in the bloodstreams of you and your children and pets.

Leonard Mehlmauer, in his *Principles of Healthy Eating*, says, "The percentage of live foods in your diet = the degree of your good health."[14] The definition of "live" varies, but Ann Wigmore said that live food was food that had been sprouted to bring forth its vital energy. Some say the energy is in the stem of the plant. At any rate, raw and/or live food will provide the body with the necessary enzymes for digestion and also the maximum amount of nutrition, in most cases. Visit websites in the appendixes to learn about the benefits of raw foods. Raw vegetables, raw nuts and seeds, and raw fruits can sustain very healthy life! Investigate sprouting and living foods. Whether vegetarian or meat eating, the source of the food is of utmost importance; the joke is on vegetarians if they aren't choosing non-GMO, organic produce and washing it well. Eating grocery store bell peppers and strawberries alone could fill the body with many poisons, making the immune system weaker and unable to handle the toxic load.

---

[13] Fitzgerald, Randall. "The Synthetics Belief System." www.hundredyearlie.com/home3. Accessed February 14, 2008.

[14] Mehlmauer, Leonard. *Principles of Healthy Eating*. Pamphlet. Found at www.grandmedicine.com.

Vegetarians Eat Vegetables!

Some people will say, "I'm a vegetarian; I only eat fish." Or, "I don't eat meat, but I eat chicken." There is no flesh-eating vegetarian. Vegetarians eat mainly vegetables by definition.

The term "vegetarian" was coined in 1847 by the founders of the Vegetarian Society of Great Britain. St. Francis of Assisi, Albert Einstein, Albert Schweitzer, H.G. Wells, Bob Barker, Benjamin Spock – the list of famous vegetarians is long.

Various sub categories have evolved over the years, including:

Vegans - Strict vegans eat only plant-based foods, excluding all flesh from animal sources (meat, fish or fowl) as well as any item made from animal products, such as dairy, eggs and honey. Many vegans also avoid animal derived by-products such as gelatin and beeswax.

Lacto Vegetarian - This diet consists of plant-based foods plus milk and products made from milk, such as cheese and yogurt. It excludes meats, fish, fowl and eggs. Many Indian families follow this plan and revere the "Mother Cow," eating not the cow but what the cow eats. They often make "curd" by pouring raw milk into boiling water; it tastes a lot like tofu; you'll see it in many Indian recipes.

Ovo Vegetarian - People following this diet eat plant-based foods plus eggs but exclude meats, fish, fowl and dairy products.

Lacto-Ovo Vegetarian - This diet includes dairy products and eggs along with plant-based foods but doesn't allow meat, fish and fowl.

The health benefit associated with eating more vegetables and fruits and less meat is pretty clear, based upon principles of acidity and alkalinity. When we consider today's sources for animal protein (feed-lot beef full of hormones and cage-raised chickens shot with steroids) becoming vegetarian is gaining in popularity.

All flesh foods are in the high acid range...remember gout was named the "rich man's disease" because only the rich could afford meat. It is, however, very hard for people eating a vegetarian diet to stay healthy if they just eat more carbohydrates and dairy, especially if they aren't watching their sources and eat refined foods. We assume that vegetarians choose better fats and eat less harmful protein than those on a standard American diet, and they consume higher levels of fiber, vitamins and minerals. Studies have shown a positive link between eating a vegetarian diet and a reduced risk for chronic diseases such as diabetes, obesity, hypertension, coronary artery disease and some types of cancer – if, vegetarians are eating properly.

Healthy Vegetarianism

That vegetarians must be super careful to choose wisely goes without saying. It is especially important for vegetarians to avoid excessive amounts of junk food since a "refined food" vegetarian diet can be potentially dangerous with its extremely low nutrient levels.

We see vegetarians who are too thin or too heavy – paying attention to variety is the key.

Vegetarians must be sure to consume enough of the right kind of calories and vegetable proteins such as sprouts, nuts and seeds along with their spinach and kale. Here is a list of alternative vegetarian sources of nutrients:

Milk – replace with fresh almond, rice or hemp milks in recipes and for drinks. Use soy sparingly because of its effect on the thyroid and the hormones.

Butter – replace with olive oil, extra virgin coconut oil or vegetable broth or water sautéing for dairy free. Use real cultured butter from organically raised, grass-fed cows or goats if you choose butters.

Cheese – use only raw, cultured cheeses. Use nut cheeses or nutritional yeast flakes. Soy, again, apparently is not the answer. It is heavily sprayed when not organic, often times genetically engineered, and may have estrogenic effects, especially for pregnant and lactating women and their children.

Legumes - eat lima beans, chickpeas, adzuki beans, lentils, black eyed peas and kidney beans.

Nuts and Seeds - almonds, pumpkin seeds, sunflower seeds, pecans, cashews, walnuts and sesame seeds.

Grains - whole and enriched grains such as quinoa, millet, spelt, brown rice.

Vegetables - all, particularly dark and leafy greens, rich yellow squash and orange, beta carotene-rich carrots.

Fresh fruits – note on the alkaline food chart that generally the sweeter the fruit, the more acidic in general, so focus on the fruits that have a more alkaline effect, such as lemons, limes, grapefruits, and watermelons.

Soy - Should you swear off tofu and throw out the soy sauce? No - for one thing, the amount of soy contained in soy sauce is comparatively low, since it consists mainly of water (sodium might be a problem, however). We just don't know; no one is sure how much soy is safe to consume. While Asians have been consuming soy for centuries, most claim that they use primarily fermented soy such as tempeh and miso. Nonetheless, since soy turns up in everything from cereal to ice cream, we may unknowingly be consuming high amounts without any real idea of the consequences. Organic sprouted tofu is now available in most grocery stores. The Westin Price Website has some excellent articles on the dangers of soy, and parents should definitely look into the issue before they use soy as a milk substitute. It is my understanding that soy infant formula has NOT been used traditionally in the Oriental countries.

What in the World Should I EAT?

In the second step, we discussed alkaline/acid balance in the blood and tissues and good fats versus bad fats. If we just stick with the 80/20 rule (80% alkaline and 20% acid foods) and avoid processed foods, we should be able to get closer to optimal health. In *The China Study*, released by Dr. Campbell, the recommendation is basically 5%-10% acid, as he recommends that protein be a maximum of 5% of the diet.

The list below is largely derived from the work of Leonard Mehlmauer in his *Principles of Healthy Eating*.

The Mainstay of Anyone's Diet

- Extra-virgin olive oil and coconut oil

- Raw and soaked nuts and seeds; peeled nuts are best.

- Sprouted nuts, seeds and grains

- Grasses such as barley, wheat grass, and alfalfa Manna and Essene type breads- sour dough

- Ezekiel sprouted tortillas and pastas have no yeast! Organic fruits and vegetables in season: raw, blended, steamed or roasted.

- Medicinal, flavorful spices such as turmeric, ginger, cinnamon and cayenne, Celtic sea salt

Eat in Smaller Amounts

- Tofu or soy substitutes – choose true veggie or bean burgers when buying convenience foods.

- Prepared mixes or boxed cereals, even organic ones from health food store

- Whole grain crackers or chips, Rice cakes, Mary's Gone Crackers, rice crackers

- Canned, stewed vegetables

- Sweeteners – honey, maple syrup, molasses, rice syrup

- Frozen yogurt and rice dream type products

- Butter and yogurt with no sugar or chemicals added

- Pickles, sauerkraut and other fermented foods Pastas of any kind

- Nut Butters

- Sprouted grain breads – Ezekiel, etc.

- Mustard, mayonnaise, unless homemade Braggs Liquid Aminos to flavor veggies, rice, eggs, pasta, etc.

(Mehlmauer calls these "health food junk foods.")

Avoid these Low-Quality Foods

- Table salt (refined sodium chloride) Any food that is not organic

- Refined foods such as flour and cornmeal, and food prepared with them

- Hydrogenated fats and oils

- Bread from commercial bakeries or made with refined grains

- Dairy products, unless raw and unpasteurized, and then sparingly

- Eggs from commercially raised chickens

- Flesh foods unless organic and grass fed, wild Alaskan, etc.

Avoid All Together

- Alcohol

- Drugs

- Smoke

Healthy Meat Eating

Proteins and fats go together metabolically. Fatty meats and whole milk products have been enjoyed by long-lived Russians in the Caucasus Mountains and in other cultures where people live unusually long lives. Dr. Bernard Jensen and other early health-conscious Americans traveled the world looking for cultures with long life and found few vegetarian cultures but instead, cultures with a varied diet and a pristine environment.

Today, a major consideration for meat eaters or vegetarians is source – what was the plant or animal fed in its lifetime. Chickens, cows, fish (including "Atlantic" salmon that are really cage raised) and sheep that have been grain fed will fatten the animal and its consumer YOU.

It is not enough to know the meat passes FDA inspection; we have to know that it was properly fed and cared for. Do slaughter houses give thanks for the animal's life before killing? Was the animal raised in a feed lot or tiny cage for its entire life and then artificially fattened to bring more profit?

Consider the following horror stories: can you trust the source of your food?

"Arsenic Widespread in Chicken, Testing Finds": The Delmarva Peninsula's 600 million chickens produce 400,000 tons of manure a year. Each full-grown chicken in a factory farm has as little as six-tenths of a square foot of space.[15]

North Carolina's 7,000,000 factory-raised hogs create four times as much waste - stored in reeking, open cesspools - as the state's 6.5 million people. Overuse of antibiotics in animals is causing more strains of drug-resistant bacteria, which is affecting the treatment of various life-threatening diseases in humans.[16]

Fifty million pounds of antibiotics are produced in the U.S. each year. Twenty million pounds are given to animals, of which 80% (16 million pounds) is used on livestock merely to promote more rapid growth. The remaining 20% is used to help control the multitude of diseases that occur under such tightly confined conditions, including anemia, influenza, intestinal diseases, mastitis, and pneumonia. The United Nations reports that all 17 of the world's major fishing areas are at or beyond their natural limits.[17]

"Researchers in Colorado have made a startling discovery. Fish, apparently male, are developing female sexual organs. Scientists believe it's the result of too much estrogen in the water and they're finding estrogen in rivers across the country." This statement made on the nightly news in 2004 has been confirmed all over the United States in cities as well as rural areas. If fish are forming male and female sex organs, what is happening to our young children today... gender confusion?

---

[15] *Study Finds Arsenic Widespread In Chicken.* Consumeraffairs.com. April 6. Accessed on January 26, 2008.

[16] Bedford, *How Our Food is Produced Matters!* AWI Quarterly, Summer, 1999.

[17] *FDA Pledges to Fight Overuse of Antibiotics in Animals.* American Medical News, February 15, 1999.

The good news is that the public is becoming aware and is demanding better food choices, evidenced in the popularity of Whole Foods stores and Fresh Markets opening up across the United States. People are willing to pay more now that they are learning the importance of organic farm methods to their health. The number of certified organic milk cows in the U.S. nearly tripled between 1992 and 1994. The United States had 537,826 certified organic laying hens in 1997, up sharply from 7,700 in 1994.[18]

Wal-Mart is, "... excited about organic food, the fastest growing category in all of food, and at Wal-Mart." CEO F. Lee Scott said, "People in all income brackets want organic food products for their family, and lower-income families should not be denied such goods due to high prices" (organicconsumers.org).

NO FAT... KNOW FAT!

CONFUSED ABOUT FATS?

Are you buying in to the "fat alarm" in America? Have you noticed that although people have been consciously consuming less saturated fat over the last thirty years, that high cholesterol is still a big problem, even bigger? Good fats play a most important role, and enough of them must play a role in our health. Omega 3 essential fatty acids are easily broken down in your body; they are found in eggs, fish, and free-range meats. They are also in flax, coconut and palm oils.

Omega 6 polyunsaturated fats are very abundant in our modern diet; in fact, there is an Omega 6 overload in this country from hydrogenated fats and vegetable oils. We now know that mono saturated fats (olive, coconut, palm, sesame) and some saturated fats as below, may actually promote health, and that

---

[18] "Animals." www.mindfully.org. Accessed January 20, 2008.

polyunsaturated fats may pose more of a real problem, mainly because we are getting too many of them in our diet from sunflower, safflower, corn, cottonseed, and soybean oils. These oils are abundant in convenience foods.

In particular, about 1/3 of the brain is saturated fat! Forty- three percent of the fat produced and stored by our bodies is saturated, and I guess if we were roasted, we would have a lot of saturated fat in us as well. Dr. Mercola mentions in his newsletters that important scientists like Linus Pauling, Mary Enig, and Uffe Ravnskov have conducted studies that show that arterial plaque is mainly made up of *refined unsaturated fats* and **not** palm, coconut, or animal saturated fat.

The bottom line is that refined, polyunsaturated vegetable fats (man-made) and fats from animals raised in feed lots are dangerous to the health of humans and animals. Get rid of them as quickly as you can. It is typical for people trying to eat healthy to say things such as, "I never eat fatty red meats, only chicken or fish," or "I don't use butter or eggs because I am watching my cholesterol." "I just use margarine or canola oil." What about, "I buy fat-free desserts and chips." UGH. What is a canola anyway? There isn't one because this oil is really from the rapeseed plant; rapeseed is used to kill insects and might be toxic to humans, too-the great "con-ola" which has duped many Americans.

When I first read about fats in Sally Fallon's cookbook, *Nourishing Traditions,* I was quite shocked, having believed vegetable oils are best. Fallon disputes what she calls "the diet dictocrats" and shows how the healthiest people on earth have included some, but not a lot, of animal protein, bone broth and animal fats such as lard and tallow in their diets.[19] It's a book worth considering. A person who chooses vegetarianism for spiritual reasons can certainly be healthy without eating animal fats, as nature has blessed us with abundant olive, coconut,

---

[19] Fallon, Sally, Pat Connolly, Mary G. Enig, Mary Enig, Ph.D. *Nourishing Traditions.* New Trends Publishers, Inc, 1999.

palm and flax oils and natural dairy to supply good fats to everyone. Most studies show vegetarians as healthier than meat eaters: they have more sustainable energy and look more youthful. Many say that in India and the Orient where many lead vegetarian lifestyles, they receive more protein than Western vegetarians because of all of the bugs and other "critters" in their food supply.

The Framingham study intrigues us. In a study done in Framingham, Massachusetts, 6,000 people were followed over several years. In the two groups studied, one ate saturated fat in high amounts; the other group ate almost none. The data showed that the ones who consumed the most saturated fat were the healthiest and usually the thinnest. The most important thing to learn from these various studies on fats is that the body needs good, digestible fats from healthy plant and animal sources, and that low fat and low cholesterol diets may not be healthier for people.

Why do you think they feed animals corn and other grains to "fatten them up?" Animals' obesity is shown to increase with unsaturated fat in their diets. When farmers fed their cows saturated coconut oil to fatten them up, the animals stayed muscular and slender. Then they tried a thyroid suppressing medication that made them gain weight but was shown to be carcinogenic, so they discontinued its use. By 1950, farmers found that corn and soybeans had the same anti-thyroid effect as the thyroid-suppressing drug, and animals could gain weight on less food.[20] Scientists found that unsaturated vegetable oils suppressed thyroid hormone. In this article, Puotenin goes on to say, "Of the popular vegetable oils, the safest is probably olive oil. However, Peat cautions, olive oils moderate content of polyunsaturated fats (about 8% to 12%), which is several times higher than that of coconut oil (usually 1% to 2%), suggests that olive oil should not be

---

[20] Puotenin, C.J. *Unhealthy Vegetable Oils? Does Food Industry Ignore Science Regarding Polyunsaturated Oils?* Article originally appeared in the Well Being Journal. Retrieved from thescreamonline.com/essays/essays5-1/vegoil.

used quite as generously as coconut oil." Ray Peat, PhD, has been studying fats for forty years. He suggests that we throw away soy, canola and corn oil as well as "tofu, soy cheese, soy yogurt, soy protein, and soy lecithin." And he adds, by the way, that we shouldn't eat commercially raised chickens or beef to get good fats because animals raised on polyunsaturated fats and their eggs or dairy products, can't provide good saturated fats – another example of "You are what you eat!"

The most important thing to remember is that fats are good for you when they are the right type of fats. In chemistry class, there was the saying that "like dissolves like," so "fats dissolve fats" might be the right way to look at this subject. How could a "no fat" diet be good for us? Mary Enig, in her article, "The Importance of Saturated Fats for Biological Functions," says the following: During the 1970s, researchers from Canada found that animals fed rapeseed oil and canola oil developed heart lesions. This problem was corrected when they added saturated fat to the animals" diets. On the basis of this and other research, they ultimately determined that the diet should contain at least 25 percent of fat as saturated fat.[21] The Weston Price website, www.westonaprice.org, has available abundant information about good fats and bad fats. Under the title, "Confused about Fats," is the following information:

The following nutrient-rich traditional fats have nourished healthy population groups for thousands of years:

- Butter
- Beef and lamb tallow
- Lard
- Coconut, palm and sesame oils
- Cold pressed olive oil
- Cold pressed flax oil or ground flax seeds

---

[21] Enig, Mary. *The Importance of Saturated Fats in Biological Functions.* The Weston A. Price Foundation Website. www.westonaprice.org/knowyourfats

- Marine oils

The following new-fangled fats can cause cancer, heart disease, immune system dysfunction, sterility, learning disabilities, growth problems and osteoporosis:

- All hydrogenated oils, including margarine and Crisco
- Soy, corn and safflower oils
- Cottonseed oil
- Canola oil

FOOD PLANS THAT WORK

Choose the food plan that fits your current condition. Always drink one ounce of water for each two pounds of body weight every day. Remember to drink a tall glass of room-temperature water each morning with lemon and cayenne to bring up your alkaline reserves, as most people are too acidic.

Plan A: Are you in good health but would like to feel better?

1. Avoid food in Category IV and V.
2. You should feel better in two weeks; if you do not, move to Food Plan B.

Plan B: Are you not feeling well and would like to lose weight?

1. Avoid food in Category III, IV, and V.
2. Eat Category I for meals.
3. Eat Category II in small amounts and only between meals.
4. If you are not better in two weeks, move to Food Plan C.

Plan C: Do you have many health problems, aches and pains or need to lose weight? If your body chemistry is in extreme need of balancing, this plan provides the most bio-available nutrients.

1. Eat only from Category I.
2. Eat one small portion from each group 5-6 times per day.

3. Continue in this category until your symptoms subside.

Plan D: For those who are ill and need to get the body back in balance. This plan will alkalize the body and is suggested as a temporary cleansing diet for those who suffer from degenerative diseases of any type.

1. Eliminate meats from Category I.
2. Continue with this program but because of its extreme limitations, supplement with green powders, smoothies, and sprouts.

Category I	Category II	Category III	Category IV
All green vegetables All root vegetables All red, yellow and orange vegetables Herbs and spices Fish Free-range Turkey Grass-fed Lean beef Free -range chickens and eggs	Most fruits other than lemons, watermelons, limes and tomatoes. Nuts other than almonds Seeds	Grains: wheat germ, white flour, whole wheat flour Pasta: Whole grain, refined spelt, or wheat Fungi: mushrooms, yeast Fruit: sweet fruits like peaches, plums, pears and grapes Nuts: pistachios and peanuts Dairy: hard and soft cheeses, milk, yogurt Miscellaneous: coffee, black tea, salt	The more consumed, the more rapid the deterioration. Alcohol Honey Cane sugar Rice syrup Beet sugar Saccharine Fructose Stevia or local honey for sweetener

Category V

These unbalance the body's chemistry: Stay away from these.

Acetaminophen	Baking powder	MSG
Aspirin	Medications	Tobacco

For the most part, this plan is not original to me. I would like to give credit to the source, but I have been unable to locate the original article as it was given to me by a friend of a friend as notes. It so matched my teaching that I adapted the concept for clients, and have used it with success.

Move to a more wholesome, cleansing diet.

Once you have accepted these changes for a six-week period, you should be free of symptoms and pain. You will be in balance; you will look and feel lively, radiant, and younger!

Use the 80-20 alkaline chart – eat what you like from the chart, but remember the ratios. Your plate will reflect this when you choose 80% fresh, water-based vegetables and only 10-20% dense carbohydrates and protein foods. Our bodies are over 70% water, so let your plate reflect this inner balance. A few recipes and some meals are included at the end of this chapter.

Stay out of the center aisles in the grocery store because all of the packaged and canned foods are there. (Canned tomatoes have been named one of the most dangerous foods in the market.) If you use canned foods, buy BPA free plastic liners and avoid aluminum linings, even in boxed foods.

Produce – choose organic. Support the produce managers by buying organic fruits and vegetables; this will encourage them to get more. When our local grocery has beautiful, organic strawberries and romaine, I call my friends so that they can support organics to keep it coming in.

Meats – First, we need to reduce consumption of animal foods because of the high protein, high acid, growth hormones, and pesticides. Demand access to free range and organic meats, limit proteins and dense foods to 20% of your daily consumption. Eat ocean-caught fish and wild Alaskan salmon.

Dairy – Again, choose organic and if your state allows it, raw dairy. Pasteurizing kills enzymes and inhibits digestion. Health food stores such as Whole Foods offer a selection of raw cheeses and, in some states, other organic, raw dairy products. Most children diagnosed with ADD, ADHD, and many other behavioral disorders greatly improve when dairy and gluten are completely removed from the diet. Substitute with organic, sprouted, almond, rice, or hemp milk.

Breads – Ask the grocer for more sprouted grain breads such as Ezekiel and Udi's gluten free products which provide better digestion and assimilation. Sprouted grains increase the vitamin and protein in the bread, and most people, even those with wheat intolerance, find they accept this style bread with no problem. Some celiac patients are able to eat sprouted breads without upsetting their digestive system.

Start building the bulk of your diet around raw choices full of enzymes and bursting with nutrition. For breakfast, choose a raw apple-spinach smoothie or sprouted grain cereal with fresh fruit and sprouted almond milk. Make a lunch plate piled high with fresh, organic greens and red and yellow vegetables. Finish the day with greens lightly sautéed in coconut oil; season with garlic, cayenne and ginger and serve over millet or quinoa (ancient grains) or some brown rice. Add almonds or other nuts. Curb your sugar addiction with fruit which is *L-Fructose,* unless you have a yeast problem; then be careful to eat more unsweet fruit.

You will want to avoid sugar for the most part – everything from desserts to cereals, breads, ketchup, and soy milk. Except for lemons, limes, grapefruits, tomatoes, and avocados, fruits contain a lot of sugar. While fruits are beautiful and have nutritional value, if you are ill, curb your intake of fruit. When you come back into balance, add fruits back as a healthy addition. Use green stevia or raw honey to sweeten, and avoid the acidic artificial sweeteners such as Splenda and Equal.

Cut back on grains, especially refined ones. First, eliminate white flour, rice, and pasta, and substitute with rice pasta, sprouted grain pasta, millet, quinoa, and spelt. Use sprouted tortillas roasted in the oven for 10-15 minutes as chips. Spray them with olive oil first, add a touch of sea salt, and then use to dip your cilantro-rich salsas and hummus. Quinoa and spelt are two ancient grains that have a more alkaline effect in the body, making them a better choice for your grain selections.

Condiments — Be aware that most condiments are acidic and loaded with sugar and sodium. Cut back on mustard, mayonnaise, and ketchup and start using olive oil, coconut, flax, and sesame oil instead. Try lemon and lime, garlic, ginger and cayenne pepper to season food. Start using more fresh and dried spices for flavor, but watch out for heavily salted mixed seasonings.

Get rid of yeast by eliminating yeast breads (yeast-free breads are available at your health food store), sugar, white vinegar, white mushrooms, peanuts and peanut butter, and alcohol. Now that may seem a lot to give up, but you will be rewarded with relief from a multitude of symptoms — everything from headaches and depression to irritable bowel syndrome. Try rice crackers and sprouted grain Ezekiel tortillas. If you love sandwiches, wrap your veggies in lettuce or nori wraps and apply whatever sauce or condiments you like. Some black bean hummus adds a rich dark protein to veggies packed into a sheet of seaweed; a good snack to eat on the go.

Make healthy snacks readily available: raw almond butter with celery or apples, sprouted tortillas, rice crackers, fresh salsa and pesto, sprouted almonds, sunflower and pumpkin seeds. Roast an assortment of veggies such as sweet potatoes, squash, onions, broccoli, and asparagus in a little coconut oil and fresh herbs. Store this mix in the fridge for healthy munching.

Drink raw smoothies at any time of day.

Once you have stocked your kitchen with these healthy choices, you will have fewer temptations to eat foods that will interfere with your health plan. Whether you are cleansing, wanting to lose unwanted pounds or reducing your chances of getting diabetes and other degenerative diseases, following the outline above will provide you with the habits and the foods you need.

Here are some healthy recipes for you to try!

PATOUT'S BREW

1 t. Granulated lecithin
Dash of cayenne
1 t. Flaxseeds
1 t. Cinnamon AND 1 t. Turmeric
1/2 - 2 c. Almond or Rice milk
Fruit (1/2 fresh, unripe banana, sour apple, watermelon, grapefruit, lemon, etc.)
And blend.

LEMON COCONUT SHAKE

C. Water or almond or rice milk
1 avocado
1 whole lemon
1 c. Spinach or broccoli (frozen is ok)
1 tsp. Stevia or Xylitol
5 tsp. Shredded coconut
2-4 tsp. Ext. Virgin coconut oil
1 scoop inner e cology or other green powder (optional)
1 handful soaked almonds or sunflower seeds

GOLDEN MILK

Heat 2 cups light, unsweetened coconut milk (or almond or soymilk)
Add 1/2 tablespoon peeled, grated fresh ginger
Add 1 tablespoon peeled, grated fresh turmeric or 1 teaspoon powder
Add 3-4 black peppercorns or 1/8 t. black pepper
Heat all ingredients in a saucepan; Stir well.
Bring to a simmer and simmer covered for 10 minutes. Stevia if desired.

CLEANSING DETOX SHAKE[22]

1 pink grapefruit

1 peeled cucumber

1 cup pineapple. Fresh cilantro

1 tsp. Coconut oil

Juice of 1 whole lemon or lime

T. Stevia and a dash of cinnamon

FRESH ALMOND MILK

Soak 1 cup organic almonds overnight in 3-4 cups clean water; pour off soaking water, add 3-4 cups more water, and blend thoroughly. Strain.

Save the pulp for muffins or dehydrated crackers. Add a pinch of celtic sea salt. To make a shake, add vanilla flavoring, stevia, or xylitol. Add a banana or other fruit (if desired) and blend.

YUMMY GREEN APPLE JUICE

Add the following to the blender:

3 or 4 ice cubes.

Sour or tart apples

T. Coconut oil

2 Handfuls organic spinach

1 Tsp. Flax seeds

2 Cups water

Stevia, honey or xylitol to taste

BASIC FUDGE

1/3 C. raw cacoa or dark cocoa powder

½ C. Extra Virgin Coconut Oil

1/3 C. Almond Butter – add honey or stevia if desired to sweeten.

Mix. Add nuts or dried fruit such as coconut, currants, or dates. Pour into molds or pour onto a plate. Refrigerate until hard. Store in fridge or freezer.

---

[22] *Going Green: The Smoothie Way* by Betty O'Brian

HOLIDAY FUDGE

1 cup rolled oats
3/4 cup carob or cocoa powder
1/4 cup sesame seeds, ground
1/4 cup sunflower seeds, ground
 1/2 cup raw almond butter
6 dates, pitted, soaked 2 hours, and drained
1/2 to 1 cup walnuts or pecans, chopped gogi berries (tart, optional)

Place all ingredients in a food processor with s blade or a blender, and mix well. Press into a lightly oiled 8" square pan. Chill, cut, and serve. Keeps in refrigerator covered for several days. Enjoy!

Organic ingredients are preferred!

Next Steps

Here are your Next Steps to clean up your diet:

☐ Pick a food plan that will work for you. Are you sick? Do you feel great? Don't challenge your body more than is necessary.

☐ Become a smart shopper and travel the outer aisles of the grocery store, stocking up on organic and free-range products.

☐ Drink at least one smoothie a day.

☐ Think about investing in a Vita Mix or a 3 HP blender, and when you do, go ahead and get a second top. Store that one under the kitchen sink, and as you increase your intake of fruits and vegetables, (and therefore plenty of peelings and scraps), make compost each evening. Just store the scraps until the end of each day, add water and blend. Broadcast or pour the liquefied scraps directly onto the lawn or into the flower beds. Instant composting!

Six Weeks to a Healthy Lifestyle

☐

Week Four: Replace Toxic Household Cleaners

"If we are going to live so intimately with these chemicals eating and drinking them, taking them into the very marrow of our bones - we had better know something about their nature and their power." Rachel Carson, Silent Spring

The goal is to rid your home of toxins which might be making your family and your pets sick. Consider making the following changes, at the very least:

☐ Take steps to remove xenoestrogens: get synthetic materials out of your closet and your indoor environment by removing carpets, using safe paints, wearing natural fiber clothes, etc.

☐ Use only natural cleaners and detergents that are biodegradable and free of dyes. Bleach and ammonia should be used sparingly, if at all. Substitute peroxide and oxygen cleaners.

☐ Check for additives such as colors, dyes, sodium laurel sulfate, alcohols, phosphates, (DEA) and mineral spirits.

☐ Support environmentally friendly companies such as those listed in this chapter and the appendix.

☐ Avoid artificial scents and sprays, including candles which may have a lead wick. Use diffusers with pure essential oils of lavender, orange, and frankincense for their healing benefits, beautiful scents, and energy clearing.

☐ Have vinegar, baking soda, peroxide, and Borax on hand in quantities suitable for making your own cleaning supplies.

☐ Investigate extreme acid (2.5) and extreme alkaline (11.5) water for disinfecting and cleaning. Save your family money and save the environment from more plastic waste by getting a water alkalizer/ionizer that separates acid and alkaline water molecules.

Substituting Healthy Alternatives for Toxic Household Cleaners

"Our house is clean enough to be healthy, and dirty enough to be happy."
Author Unknown

If your home or office is typical, it already has dozens of cleaning and personal care products that contain harmful chemicals in addition to the varnishes, synthetic fabrics and carpets, plastic window blinds, and polyurethane coated floors. Most homes and offices contain dangerous products that may harm or kill your children and you. We have all heard family horror stories about a child drinking poison... what if their poison is coming in more slowly from furniture polish, carpet fresheners, dryer sheets and bleach?

Some of us have learned of the dangers in a toxic home by suffering the consequences and tracing the cause directly to home environment, at least in part. One client developed huge swelling in the breasts, lumps that were painful to the touch, and the gynecologist had no explanation other than that she must have an estrogen overload. She was not taking any estrogen or other hormone medications or supplements. We were able to trace it back to her home remodeling; she had chosen an inexpensive synthetic carpet and paneling to close in her garage a month earlier. Each day, she was spending many hours in the room painting and then using it as an art studio. Once we realized that the chemical overload was causing xenoestrogens to overload her hormone system, she began drinking red clover tea to fill up those receptors with a safer estrogen, used castor oil packs with heat on her breasts, and stayed out of the addition. Within a week, the inflammation was gone, but unfortunately, the toxic room was still there.

Eliminate some of the toxic chemicals in the home by making thoughtful choices in the supermarket. According to a new study by researchers at the University of California, Berkeley, and Lawrence Berkeley National Laboratory, "When used indoors under certain conditions, many common household cleaners and air fresheners emit toxic pollutants at levels that may lead to health risks."[23] No kidding! This is old news to most of us, but old habits die hard, as they say, and it is easier to continue polluting the earth with Tide and Dawn than it is to convert to a new way of thinking about cleaning your home and office.

This plumbing story reveals the dangers of commercial laundry detergents. Shortly after we moved into a house raised up on piers, the plumbing under the washing machine started leaking, and my husband made a temporary drain that led from the washer to a flower bed in the front yard. After a week of Cheer detergent in the laundry water, all of the beautiful azaleas in that bed began to wither and shed their leaves. When I saw, what was happening, I changed to a biodegradable detergent and a little peppermint oil; immediately the plants started to recover.

Now just imagine what is happening to our Mother Earth as Tide, Cheer, Fab and whatever detergents are flowing by the millions of gallons into her. We see her rebelling in every way that she can, trying to push us into using products that the earth can recycle instead of products that are completely choking her — could this relate to tsunamis, hurricanes, tornados, and

---

[23] Greensfelder, Liese. *Study Warns of Cleaning Product Risks.* UC Berkeley News . www.berkeley.edu/news/media/releases/2006. Accessed February 1, 2008.

earthquakes? I believe that the earth will survive – with or without us. Some of what happens is in our hands, especially when it comes to our own households. If you take nothing else away from this chapter, RECYCLE, and do your part in the little things – less plastic, glass for storage in the refrigerator, take your own bag to the market, shop local, etc. Greenpeace was out there blowing up whaling ships. That kind of crazy - major action might trickle down to our becoming conscious consumers and affecting the earth in the best way we can.

Another devilish household product that will adversely affect your pets and your children is carpet freshener. I discovered this one when my dog kept developing hot spots on his skin that no amount of creams, ointments, or baths (or fewer baths) would help. One day, I was at home when the cleaning ladies came armed with a commercial carpet-fresh type product that they had purchased at the dollar store. They said that they wanted the house to smell good when I arrived home, and that this was the most "lingering" scent they could find. After reading the ingredients, I asked them not to use it anymore, and all of my dog's hot spots were gone for good. Now, if it puts hot spots on animals, what might it be doing to crawling infants or young children playing on the floor? Just think about it!

Once you have acquired the knowledge, you are fore-armed to enter the market as an educated consumer. If you want to know what toxins are in your home, take a look at these household cleaners lurking in your cabinets at home. You may have a small fortune invested in them, but if you take 30 minutes to clean out your cabinets (no, don't give them to a shelter – send them to the hazardous waste disposal collections), you and your family will breathe easier and experience greater health.

Trisodium nitrilotriacetate is found in laundry detergents and can disrupt waste water treatment.

Chlorine bleach (sodium hypochlorite) is found in the fatty tissues of wild animals and is toxic to all animals that live in the water or soil.

Phosphates, also an ingredient in dishwasher and laundry detergents, cause algae bloom and creates a chemical that is toxic to humans and animals that unknowingly drink the water.

Formaldehyde is found in furniture polish and baby shampoo![24]

"Thirty years ago, the major childhood illnesses were chickenpox, measles and mumps. Now they are asthma, ADD/ADHD, Autism Spectrum, and Cancer – most of which have been linked to chemicals in the home."[25]

So Where Will You Find These Dangerous Chemicals?

In the Kitchen and Bathroom:

All-purpose cleaner, ammonia-based cleaners, bleach, brass or other metal polishes, dishwater detergent, disinfectant, drain cleaner, floor wax or polish, glass cleaner, dishwashing detergent, oven cleaner, and scouring powder contain dangerous chemicals.

It's a good idea to switch to a natural, environmentally friendly product lines like Shaklee or Ecover and to keep the following common household products available. You can make your own cleaners with a little lemon, vinegar and baking soda. Consider some of these uses of products you already have in the cabinet at home for your staples:

---

24 Mitchell,Deborah. *Switch to Natural Cleaning Products.* www.charityguide.org. Accessed October 20, 2007.
25 Nelson, Debi. *To Clean Or Not To Clean.* Freeinfozone.com. Accessed January 30, 2008.

- Baking Soda – laundry powder, abrasive cleaner, deodorizer.
- Vinegar or lemon – for countertops, glass, drain cleaner, brass and copper cleaner.
- Peroxide and acid water (2.5 pH) – as disinfectants.

Many of the cleaners listed below have been taken directly from a government website that is full of information about natural lifestyles: www.noaa.gov. These are well-known natural alternatives.

Laundry Detergent: Use 1-2 scoops of baking powder (large bucket at Sams) and add Dr. Bronner's Peppermint oil castile soap or essential oil of lavender, peppermint, orange or lemon for scent if wanted. Borax and peroxide or an oxygen cleaner may be used to boost the whitening.

Oven Cleaner -Avoid the use of harsh chemicals by wiping away grease and spills after use. For spills, let oven cool slightly, sprinkle salt on the spill, wait a few minutes and wipe area clean with a wet cloth. For scouring the oven, use baking soda (do not let baking soda touch wires or heating elements) and a damp sponge. Scour racks and burner inserts with steel wool.

Drain Cleaner- Chemical drain cleaners are among the most dangerous of all cleaning products. Most contain corrosive ingredients such as sodium hydroxide and sodium hypochlorite (bleach) that can permanently burn eyes and skin. Some can be fatal if ingested.

For clogged drains, try a plunger first. Dissolve 4 ounces baking soda and 8 oz. vinegar in a small amount of boiling water. Pour down drain and wait for fizzing to stop. Flush with tap water.

Toilet Bowl Cleaner -Sprinkle baking soda around the bowl followed by vinegar. Scrub with a toilet brush. Vinegar is a mild acid and should remove hard water scale.

Abrasive Powder Cleansers -Sprinkle any of the following on the surface to be cleaned: baking soda, borax, or dry table salt and scour with a damp sponge. Rinse thoroughly with water to remove grit.

Basin, Tub, and Tile Cleaner -Cut a lemon in half and dip it in borax. Rub surfaces with lemon and rinse.

Ceramic Tile Cleaner -Mix 1/4 cup vinegar in 1 gallon of water. Scrub with a brush. Oxygen cleaners work beautifully for tile.

Mildew Remover -Dissolve 1/2 cup vinegar and 1/2 cup borax in warm water. Apply to tiles and grout with a sponge or brush. Wipe and rinse clean.

Window cleaner -Mix a solution of 2 tablespoons vinegar to 1 quart water. Apply with a wad of newspaper.

Dishwasher Soap- Mix 1 part borax and 1 part baking soda. Depending on how hard the water is, adjust proportions to avoid soap film on dishes.

Carpet stains – Use oxygen cleaners and/or Shaklee Basic H. Blot spills.

Furniture Polish: Watch out for polishes. Furniture polish can be flammable and dangerous because most brands contain petroleum distillates – very dangerous if swallowed or if the hands come in contact with the mouth after using such polishes. The aerosol spray polishes damage lung tissue and some contain formaldehyde.

Mix 1 part lemon juice with 2 parts olive or vegetable oil or mix 2 teaspoons lemon oil and 1 pint mineral oil in a spray bottle.

Stain Removal – Often times a little water and biodegradable soap will remove the stains, especially if the cloth is set in the direct sun for about 15-30 minutes.

Most people have heard the reports on antibacterial soaps, such as the Liquid Dial bathroom soaps. Disinfectants might kill germs on the surface, but they don't provide any lasting disinfection. Alkylphenol ethoxylates found in many of these soaps disrupt hormones and are not biodegradable. When these go down your drain, they end up threatening fish and other wildlife in our rivers and streams. In a study conducted by the U.S. Geological Survey, triclosan, which is found in many anti-bacterials, was found in 57.6% of U.S. water samples taken from across the United States.[26] No one wants to allow E. coli bacteria or salmonella to survive in the food supply, but we can't let our fear of germs cause even more problems for the ailing earth. Washing hands with a good castile soap and using vinegar and lemon or citric acid to disinfect the hands will not only help the environment, it will keep you and your family in better health, as the good bacteria just might survive such a sensible method of control.

Thieves oil and spray from Young Living Oils is one of the most fantastic anti-bacterials available, and it is completely safe for the environment.

Air Fresheners: Spritz the air with lavender water or any citrus essential oil. Clean the air by opening windows and using fans on days that the weather allows. Every morning, open the door to allow in the early morning air. Everyone knows that baking soda removes odors from the refrigerator and from the air as well, so put out little saucers of cedar scented soda or salt. The crystals used as deodorant mentioned in Week One are available specifically for refrigerator odors. Pieces of cedar and sachets of dried roses or rosemary will provide a gentle and lasting fragrance. Avoid oils and potpourri that list "artificial

---

[26] *Alternatives to Household Hazards.* Appendix.
www.yoto98.noaa.gov/books/clncoast/append1.htm. Accessed January 3, 2008.

fragrance" as an ingredient, and use only pure essential oils from a company such as Young Living, Doterra or Nature's Sunshine which are widely available on the internet.

Bug Killers: Diatomaceous Earth is ground fossilized shells and will kill all types of bugs, including fleas, ants, etc., and it won't hurt us or our pets.

Mosquitoes: 10 to 20 drops essential oil, 2 T. vegetable oil, Aloe Vera mixed with some of the following: Pennyroyal, lemon balm (citronella), thyme, lavender, sassafras, lavender, eucalyptus, pennyroyal, cedar, lemon balm (citronella), and peppermint

Roaches: Plain boric acid helps, but some of these other mixtures might be more effective. Some recipes say to add flour, and grated onions with water to bind it into a paste.

If you are not interested in making your own cleaners out of common household ingredients, you might want to consider just going natural. You will save the environment and a great deal of money through the years. A number of all-purpose cleaners that are gentler on human health and the environment are becoming more widely available in conventional grocery and home stores, but many can be found only at natural foods stores or must be ordered by mail. See Appendix A for a list of suppliers.

Water ionizers are becoming widely available now; these machines can separate water molecules into alkaline (drinking and cleaning) water and acid (disinfecting) water. The acid water makes amazing germ-eliminating cleaner. Use super alkaline (11.5) pH in place of laundry detergent. For each load of laundry, add 3-4 cups of alkaline water; use essential oils or a capful of Dr. Bronner's peppermint soap or lemon essential oil to add a scent, if desired.

My husband brought home mildewed cushions from the farm. These yellow cushions were black all around the edges and grey in the middle. He washed them twice with bleach, detergent and hot water. The cushions were still black. I poured a bucket of 11.5 pH water and put the cushions in to soak overnight with no detergent. Imagine his surprise when I pulled them out of the bucket the next morning completely clean and bright yellow, with no evidence of the mildew!

Next Steps

Here are your Next Steps to clean up your home:

☐ Check your cabinets, your closets and your carpets for synthetics. Begin to get off of the "slippery slope" and get Green!

☐ Check your laundry room and kitchen pantry for hazardous chemical cleaners. Use them as quickly as you can or, better yet, take them to a hazardous waste disposal site.

☐ Convert gradually to bio-friendly products that will help save Mother Earth (and your family).

☐ Invest in the basics of baking soda, salt, and vinegar. Use these and a little elbow grease to clean almost anything.

☐ Open your house up to outdoor air so that you let some of the fumes from synthetics escape.

☐ Use green paints and natural fabrics when possible.

Week Five: Understand Energy Healing

"The wind blows where it wishes, and you hear its sound, but you do not know where it comes from or where it goes. So it is with everyone who is born of the Spirit." – John 3:8

- ☐ Begin to understand life as energy instead of just chemistry.

- ☐ Regulate your chi through chakra balancing, acupressure, acupuncture, flower essences, meditation, yoga, reflexology, etc.

- ☐ Investigate Reiki, Healing Touch, The Reconnection and other energy techniques.

- ☐ Learn about the Optimatrix: Iridology, Sclerology, Rayid, and Time Risk Iridology. Study the eye to learn about your physical and emotional health.

- ☐ Try meditation for its healing effects on the physical, mental and emotional body

- ☐ Sound healing might supply the missing link to your health problems; what if a missing musical note would supply what your health has been missing, bringing your body into harmony?

Energy Healing

"I'm that, you're that, all this is that, and that's all there is... " ancient Vedic wisdom

I often think about how lucky we are to be living in the time of energy medicine, no longer bound by the constrictions of the conventional medical model. It frees us to know that healing takes place on many levels – the subtle body (energy body) and the physical body, and it makes us more responsible for our well-being to know that our thoughts and emotions actually correlate to our health.

One of the pioneers in the exploration of how our thoughts affect our health, Caroline Myss, explores many cases of emotional imbalances in the chakra system that create specific types of illnesses. (*The Anatomy of the Spirit*, Myss) We see this same idea reflected in the entire new energy medical model.

In *A Practical Guide to Vibrational Medicine*, Dr. Gerber compares this new view to the conventional view as follows:

Conventional Medicine	Vibrational Medicine
Based on Newtonian Physics	Based on Einsteinian and Quantum Physics
Views the body as a biomachine	Views the body as dynamic energy system
Sees the brain as a biocomputer with consciousness as part of the brain's electrical system	Mind and Spirit are true sources of consciousness
Emotions thought to influence illness through neuro-hormonal connections between brain and body	Emotions and spirit can influence illness via energetic and neuro-hormonal connections among body, mind, and spirit.
Treatments with drugs and surgery to fix abnormal bio-mechanisms in the physical body	Treatment with different forms and frequencies of energy to rebalance body/ mind /spirit complex

Instead of viewing health through the germ theory, the new view sees the complex energetic make-up of the physical, acknowledging the impact of negative emotions, thoughts, acceptance and attraction. We used to hear the expression stress kills, but now we know that it really does: stress, consciousness, and our attitudes towards life have as much to do with who gets an illness as the existence of a germ or virus or bacteria.[27] Some of the new paradigm in medicine is rediscovering what ancient healers knew, but awareness of quantum thought is magnifying our use of vibrational medicine rapidly. With so much knowledge available to us through the internet and the media, people can leave the doctor's office and literally, within minutes, be reading about people who have been saved from some dread disease through the use of Reiki, chakra healings, energy healings, healing touch, sound therapy... ideas unheard of in modern, popular culture until this century.

As an iridologist and sclerologist, I have learned that everything in nature has a vibration, and that the vibrations in the iris of the eye connect to the organs and tissues of the body and of the very essence of the person. If certain vessels of the iris are raised and white (high vibration), then the corresponding internal tissues are acutely affected by the hyperactivity (over-acidity). The same applies to dark areas in the iris; a darker or thinner area in the iris reflects a slower vibration, indicating some weakness in that area.

---

[27] Gerber, Richard. *A Practical Guide to Vibrational Medicine.* New York: Harper Collins Publishers, Inc. 2000.

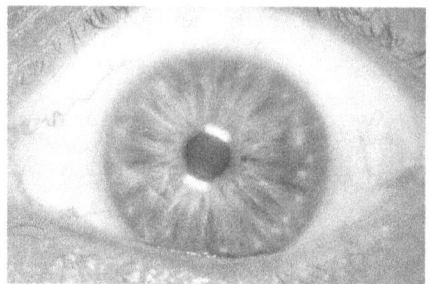

Raised, white fibers indicate overactivity; in this picture, we see bright white dots on the periphery (lymph activity) and some white fibers radiating outward toward them, indicating "hot spots" or spots needing to be calmed or nourished.

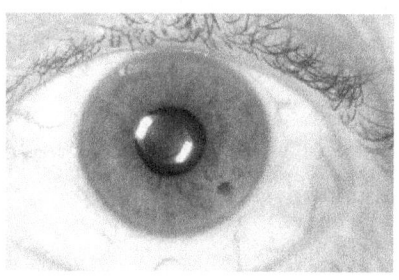

The dark pigment in the lower right and the tiny football shape over it would indicate a "cold spot" or an area that needs tonic nutrition. We want to nourish and build up such an area.

Every week someone walks into my office and says something such as, "I've got to get my life back. I've been prescribed antibiotics and two inhalers, but I feel worse after three rounds." These people are usually more committed to working a program of diet and exercise, working with an EFT therapist (Emotional Freedom Technique), receiving spinal adjustments from a physical therapist or a chiropractor, and are open to energy healings of any sort. When what we are doing is not working, sometimes accepting responsibility for our choices just makes sense and asking for referrals to others is your right.

Recently, in announcing a new gym complex, Dr. David McAfee - founder and president of the e-Fitness Center had this to say: "This center is truly a balance between mind, body and spirit because that's what creates wellness. A pill is not the answer. Changing the person's physiology is the answer.[28]

---

[28] McAfee, David, M.D. "Wellness Done Well." Sun Herald. C-7. December 6, 2007.

We are living in the 21st century, the century of energy medicine. Developing an understanding of how and why this line of reasoning might be beyond current, established scientific thought will benefit all of us.

If you want to understand why ancient healing methods work, look to humankind's most modern science: quantum physics. Wave-particle duality, the properties of electromagnetic fields, the holographic effect, the impact of the observer - these discoveries can help explain how homeopathy cures, why the holistic approach is so effective, how Reiki and Qigong can heal tissues, what makes iridology an effective diagnostic tool, and why placebos work over thirty percent of the time.

For many years, we have had the tools to test alternative therapies and show that they work. But because we never had the scientific understanding to explain why they work, we pretended they didn't.

Remember this when your doctor tells you something is "unscientific." *He may mean simply that the science he has learned is not advanced enough to explain it.* Quantum science may explain it, but doctors are not required to take that class - yet.[29]

This book offers only a brief overview of some aspects of energy healing. Please explore these books on these subjects. They are all worth your investigation.

- Gerber, Richard. *A Practical Guide to Vibrational Medicine.* New York: Harper Collins Publishers, Inc. 2000.
- Barnard, Julian. *Bach Flower Remedies.* Lindisfarne Books, 2004.
- Pearle, Eric. *The Reconnection.* Carlsbad: Hay House, 2001. 8.Trivieri, Larry Jr. Health on the Edge. New York: Penguin, 003.

---

[29] Tsalaky, Teresa. *Traditional Healing Meets Modern Science.* AAHA Self Help Articles. December 8, 2008. www.ahha.org/articles. Accessed January 5, 2008.

Have you seen the movies What the Bleep Do We Know? and The Secret? These two movies reveal certain metaphysical truths that are universal laws of nature and emphasize the idea that we really do influence the creation of our own reality, or at least our own experience of it. If you want to understand the source of the secret, visit Abraham Hicks on Youtube. After listening to several of these recordings, you'll know where she got "the secret."

"Thoughts are things."

"What we can conceive, we can achieve." (Think and Grow Rich by Napolean Hill)

In a recent Family Circus comic, the grandmother said to Billy, "You know, Billy, you are not what you think you are. But what you think... you are."

And even in the Holy Bible: "As a man thinketh in his heart, so is he." Proverbs 23:7.

To sum up this idea, in a quantum world, we are all made of the same stuff, and we are connected to everyone and everything in the universe. When Jesus said to love your neighbor as yourself, he meant that you are your neighbor, and as you love yourself, so will you love your neighbor, and vice versa. By sending out peaceful thoughts and energies, we become peaceful. By having loving thoughts, we become love. And so it is.

Another topic to explore is the exciting field of epigenetics; we are learning that it is not only our thoughts and experiences that influence our emotional and physical health, it is the traumas and unresolved issues of our ANCESTORS that are affecting us today! Soon we should learn how to protect our children from the inheritance of our anger patterns or insecurities by learning how to connect with our grandparents! Download the "Global Gratitude" booklet to get started; you'll find it on Google or www.rayid.com.

The Chakra System

In energy medicine, the Aura surrounds the body's field and when fully functioning, it can be four or five feet across. It has at least seven major layers surrounding the physical body and is basically powered by the seven chakras. The chakras are the body's seven main energy centers. The word "chakra" is derived from the Sanskrit and literally means wheel; some sources refer to it as an energy vortex. These chakras are associated with the consciousness but manifest their state of balance or imbalance through the physical body. While we can't usually see them, we can see their effects when different health issues surface in the body.

The Seven Chakra Centers and their locations in the Body:

Root or base chakra – red. Located at the base of the spine.

Naval or sacral plexus chakra – orange. Lower abdomen.

Solar plexus chakra – yellow. Below the chest but above the navel.

Heart chakra – green. In the heart center of the chest.

Throat chakra – light blue. The throat

Brow chakra – dark blue or indigo. Between the eyebrows.

Crown chakra – white or violet. Slightly above the head.

Martin Brofman's chart of **Chakra Man[30]**; showing the energy fields surrounding the physical body and the chakras within the body on the next two pages..

---

[30] Brofman, Martin, Ph.D. "Chakra Reference Chart." The Brofman Foundation for the Advancement of Healing. www.healer.ch/Chakras-e. Accessed May, 2005.

STRUCTURE

Yang   CAUSAL BODY
Male   BUDDHIC (NIRVANIC) BODY
Will   ETHERIC BODY
Acting   ASTRAL BODY
                   MENTAL BODY
             EMOTIONAL BODY
               PHYSICAL BODY

Vibrations	Nerves	System
Musical Notes	Glands	Elements
Violet	Brain	Nervous System
B Si	Pineal	Inner Light
Indigo	Carotid Plexus	Growth, Endocrine System
A La	Pituitary	Inner Sound
Blue	Cervical Plexus	Metabolism
G Sol	Thyroïd	Ether
Green	Cardiac Plexus	Respiration, Circulation, Immune System
F FA	Thymus	Air
Yellow	Solar Plexus	Skin, Muscles, Digestive System
E Mi	Pancreas	Fire
Orange	Lombar Plexus	Assimilation and Reproduction
D Re	Gonads	Water
Red	Sacral Plexus	Skeleton, Lymph, Elimination System
C Do	Adrenals	Earth

EXPERIENCE

(Deepest Inner Experience)
CAUSAL BODY — Yin
BUDDHIC (NIRVANIC) BODY — Female
ETHERIC BODY — Spirit
ASTRAL BODY — Feeling
MENTAL BODY
EMOTIONAL BODY
PHYSICAL BODY
(Outermost Level of Experience)

God
White Light
Father

Sense

Area of Consciousness

Soul — Empathy

Unity
Universal Consciousness
Source of Direction and Intuition

Spirit — Extra Sensory Perception

Spiritual Awareness
Individualized Consciousness

Hearing

Expressing, Receiving, Abundance
Flowing Manifestation
Listening to Intuition

Touch

Relating, Giving
Perceptions of Love
Acceptance

Having

Personality — Vision

Freedom/Power
Controle, Self-Definition
Intellect

Taste

Sensations
Feeling & Feelings
Food, Sex, Appetite

Smell

Safety, Security
Trust - Survival
Money, Home, Job

Mother Earth

The various charts in this chapter reveal how the eyes, the hands, the feet, and even the teeth correlate to the glands, organs, and tissues in the body. Understanding this information can help us understand the overall health of an individual and can pinpoint which chakra areas are out of balance. Herbs, flower essences, Reiki, and healing touch help us bring the energy center back into balance and can pave the way to healing.

Sometimes one EFT (Emotional Freedom Technique) or energy treatment can reverse a chronic health issue. Just as the heart pumps blood through the veins and arteries, the chakras act as valves that control how energy flows through the body.4All color has a frequency or a vibration that matches the color. The frequencies of the lower chakras, which relate to our survival in the physical world, are lower than the higher chakras, which relate to the heart and the intuition and the spirit.

Optimatrix© – the Arts of the Eye: Iridology, Sclerology, Rayid, and Time Risk

I like to call iridology and sclerology "God's Little MRI." A wealth of information presents itself in the iris and sclera of the eye – such information has been known for thousands of years. Ancient cultures from China to Egypt studied the eye to reveal health. One interesting correlation is with the Egyptian symbol for the Eye of Horus (seen above), believed to have healing and protective properties and pharmacists' formulations of prescriptions: the symbol Rx.

Sclerology, the analysis of the white sclera of the eye, has also evolved for hundreds of years. American Indians seem to have always known about sclerology and used it to diagnose health problems; it is my understanding that Dr. Stuart Wheelwright learned sclerology from the Indians and refined the charts that are still in use today. Dr. Wheelwright, whose life story can be read in *New Dimensions In Herbal Healing* by Dr. Jack Tips, founded Systemic Formulas. On the next page is a copy of one of Dr. Tips' chart showing a map of the white of the eye; yes, those bloodshot eyes really do mean something. They mean a great deal. A red line running across the sclera is an indicator of which tissues might be stressed in the body. A certified sclerologist can help interpret these signs in the sclera.

The eye as a tool for analysis will establish itself in the future as invaluable as it can reveal health issues, levels of health and constitutional weaknesses. Much work is being done in medical and alternative communities around the world. In the United States, Dr. Bernard Jensen kept the practice and study of Iridology alive even as herbalists and alternative healers were being harassed, punished, and even arrested for trying to help people in a natural way. Thank goodness for his persistence, for today we have organizations such as the International Iridology Practitioners' Association, the American College of Iridology and the Sclerology Institute that are helping to raise the standards and to certify people who are intrigued and fascinated by God's Little MRI (Iridology).

Sclerology and Iridology Charts

Many people have designed charts to guide an analysis of the sclera (white) and the iris (colored area) of the eyes. The sclerology chart below is followed by an energy iridology chart based upon the chakra system. Both charts are best viewed in color and can be ordered through the author at www.iridologyacademy.org or www.southerninstituteofnaturalhealth.com.

The sclerology chart below is based upon the work of A. Stuart Wheelwright and was produced by Dr. Jack Tips, Director of the Sclerology Institute. Imagine, as you inspect the chart, that you are seeing the red lines in the white of your eyes projected into the specific areas defined on the chart. You might want to hold the chart in front of you as you look into the bathroom mirror to find areas of stress in the body. The closer the marks are to the iris, the more imminent the concerns.

The two charts that follow offer a guide to the iris correlating to the chakras. Oftentimes, an iridologist or sclerologist is able to pinpoint emotional issues and how they are affecting the physical body (and vice versa) by weaknesses that show up in these various energy centers.

Marks such as spots, flower petal shapes, or raised white or light fibers in the lower chakras indicate issues in the physical body having to do with survival and decision making surrounding family, money, housing, jobs, etc. Marks in the upper chakras (from the heart or Chakra 4) up, relate to matters of love, intuition, spirit and the higher self.

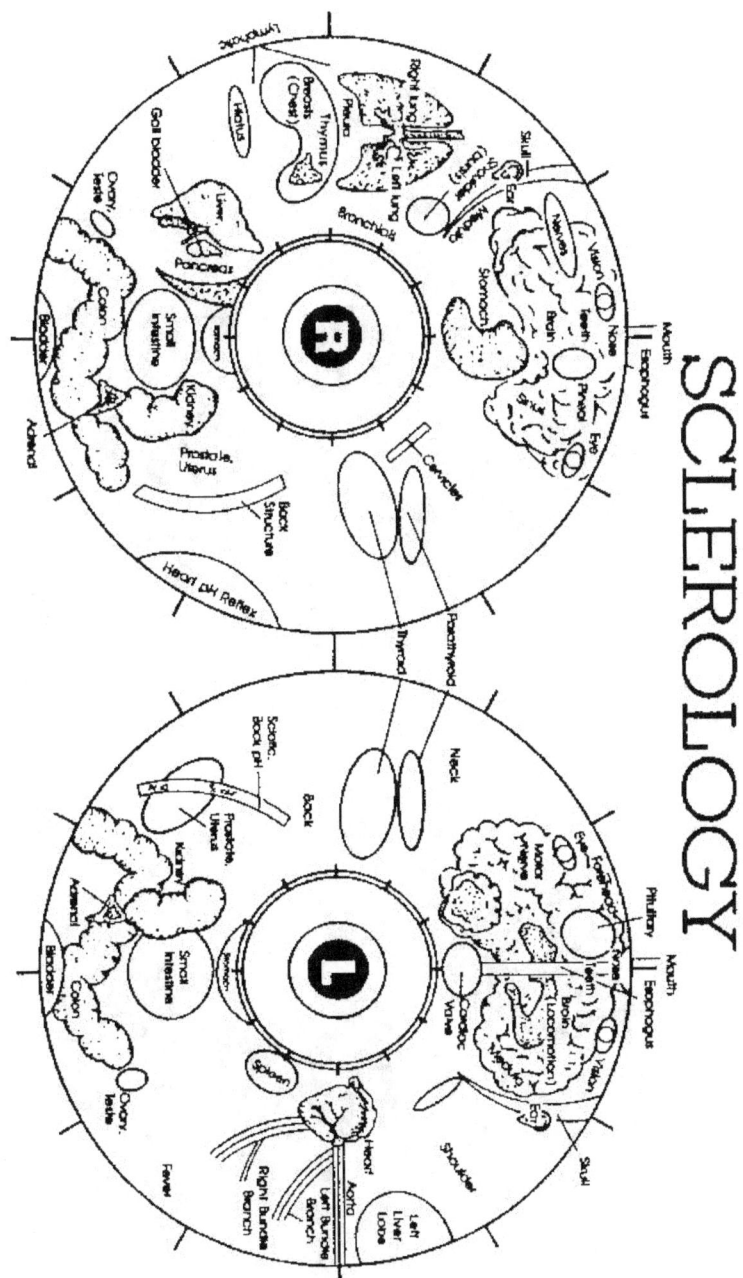

SCLEROLOGY

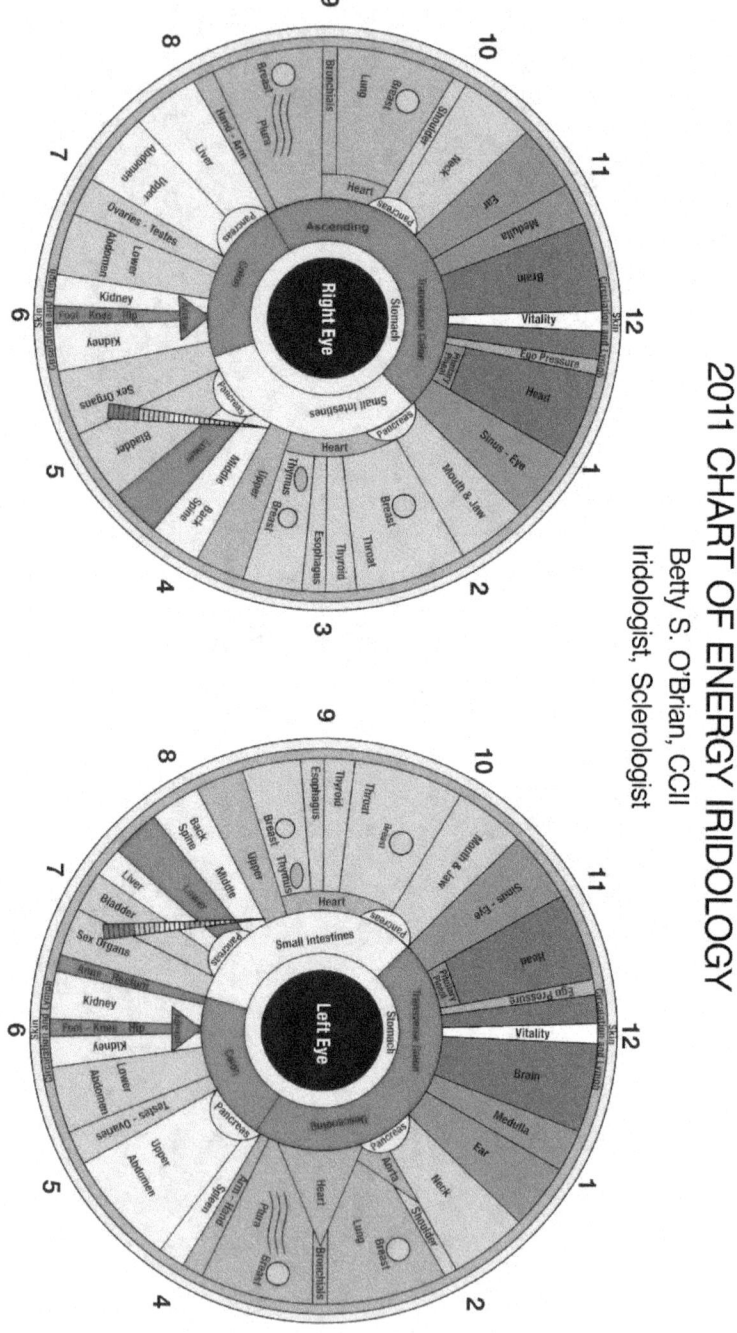

2011 CHART OF ENERGY IRIDOLOGY
Betty S. O'Brian, CCII
Iridologist, Sclerologist

Chakras (Sanskrit for "wheel")

7th chakra Lesson: "Release the past." Understanding.

Purple; White Light; "SILENCE"

Center of consciousness, nervous, muscular, skeletal and skin

6th chakra Lesson: "Learning from mistakes." Intuition.

Indigo; Inner Light; the sound "OM"

Cognition, brain, nervous system, eyes, ears, pineal, pituitary, nose

5th chakra Lesson: "Give personal will to the divine." Communication.

Blue; Ether; the sound "HAM"

Throat, thyroid, neck, mouth, teeth and gums, swollen glands

4th chakra Lesson: "Love and Divinity." Love.

Green; Air: the sound "YAM"

Heart, blood, circulation, lungs, chest, respiration, thymus, arms and hands, breast, lymph, muscle

The upper chakras relate to the higher self. Energy.

3rd chakra Lesson: "Honor yourself."

Yellow; Fire; the sound "RAM

Digestion, abdomen, upper intestines, stomach, liver, gallbladder, pancreas, mid-spine, kidney, spleen

2nd chakra Lesson: "Honor others." Emotion.

Orange, Water; the sound "VAM"

Reproduction, lower intestines, bladder, appendix, hips

1st chakra Lesson: "We are all one." Survival.

Red; Earth: the sound "LAM"

Low back, varicose veins, adrenal glands, immune disorders, excretion, legs and feet

One recent example was a female client whose whole fourth chakra area (as revealed in the iris near 3 o'clock and 9 o'clock) was covered with lacuna (shapes) and pigments (colored spots); both of these indicate potentially weaker conditions in a specific area (the lung and breasts). In addition, she had red lines in the sclera pointing to the same areas. When asked about her breasts, she confirmed that she had fibrocystic breasts and had had several biopsies of the left (mother) breast, but all had been benign. Well, the breasts are our area of nurturing, mothering, and love. When I asked her about her relationship with her mother, she said, I hate her; I resent her for never being there for me. She actually left me with a relative for months at a time, and to this day, she has only said she loved me once. She also told me that her mother and her maternal grandmother both had died of breast cancer and that they both had heart problems (also in the 4th chakra area) as well.

Gaining information such as this in a short session with a client will help to pinpoint the cause of the illness and may provide enough information to break the pattern of anger and resentment, both known to be contributors to cancer and to heart disease. As for this client, we suggested healing herbs for the breasts such as saw palmetto and red clover and rosemary. She was referred to an Emotional Freedom Technique practitioner, and we used *Emotion Code* to release some of the patterns of anger. We also worked on forgiveness through prayer work with her grandmothers. Although deceased, they still held a powerful grip on her emotional and physical health. Today this client is steadily improving through good nutrition and energy work. It is more and more apparent that the patterns in the family tree deepen through each generation and cause health problems until the pattern of anger or hatred is gone.

An angry father who belittles his son because his father did the same will create liver problems in future generations. A wonderful young man came to see me with several complaints: a pionidal cyst, which is a cyst at the bottom of the tailbone (coccyx) that can become infected and filled with pus, a hydrocele, a collection of fluid around the testicle, and an abdominal hernia. It was obvious that all of these conditions were centered in the first and second chakra areas. When I asked him about his relationship with his parents, he said that his father had basically abandoned him emotionally when his parents divorced. While the young man seemed to long for a relationship, the father made no overtures. The first and second chakras relate to our feelings of support from our families and community and feelings of self-worth energetically. He made an appointment with a Brennan energy healer and had a good result. The energy worker knew nothing of his experience with his father, but said after the treatment that every time she tried to work on this young man, the male presence of his father seemed to appear, almost trying to interfere with the session. Today, he is happily married and has no more signs of his earlier physical problems as far as we know.

The iris chart reflects the chakra system and how the chakras are revealed in the physical body; once we have this information we know which chakra to support. This is readily confirmed through muscle testing.

Two newer developments in studies of the iris include the work of pioneers Danielle LoRito from Italy and Denny Johnson of the USA who founded Time Risk Iridology and Rayid. Both of these studies are invaluable to anyone who wants to help others through the iris. In Time Risk, the practitioner studies the collarette, also called the autonomic nerve wreath, to discover information about the nervous system and the emotional causes of dis-ease in the body. With this experimental work, traumas in a person's life can be discovered and healed through the proper nurturing techniques and herbal nervous system support. In Johnson's Rayid, personality types are studied through the structural patterns in the iris. This is deep and profound work which must be studied seriously; it continues to be developed through the efforts of Denny Johnson and his guides. The best introduction to Rayid is through his website www.rayid.com or through his writings, especially his landmark book, *What the Eye Reveals*. You can study basic Rayid at www.iridologyacademy.org.

Muscle Testing

If you are not familiar with muscle testing, read the book *Power Vs Force* by David Hawkins or *Touch for Health* by John Thie, D.C. Muscle testing (applied kinesiology) uses the body's own energy to evaluate imbalances or weaknesses such as organ weaknesses, food allergies, nutritional needs, and other information. Dr. Hawkins tested words, concepts, and beliefs and worked with thousands of people to see how their bodies reacted just to holding a substance near their bodies. Applying some pressure to a muscle such as the arm or hand while a person is holding an herb, vitamin or supplement will reveal whether that substance is making the person stronger or weaker. One amazing result he got was when he wrote names on two slips of paper and put them in sealed envelopes; on one was the name Abraham Lincoln and on the other was written Adolph Hitler. One hundred percent of the time, people tested weak on Hitler and strong on Lincoln, EVEN WHEN THEY DIDN'T KNOW WHAT WAS WRITTEN ON THE PAGE!

One of the important aspects to muscle testing is polarity; if a person's energy is somehow blocked, he or she might be doing everything right, taking herbs, getting massages, being adjusted, eating alkaline yet staying sick with something such as fibromyalgia, lupus, multiple sclerosis, or other common degenerative diseases. Sometimes, until the polarity is unblocked or reset, the client will not improve and will develop chronic health issues. I usually try to get the person to drink water to ensure that they are not dehydrated. Other useful means for getting the energy balanced include drinking liquid chlorophyll or taking spirulina or alfalfa supplements and tapping the "sore spot," a spot about three inches down from the sternum and three inches to the left. Usually after a short while on the green supplements, a person's balance is back; while out of balance, herbs, supplements and other treatments seem to have no effect. Many clients who have been chronically overweight become balanced when put on spirulina for a few months, and their weight comes into balance. This seems like an oversimplification of a complex issue, but often there are simple solutions to difficult scenarios. Keith Smith in Escondido, CA, has worked with polarity for many years; in *The Indigo Children*, he explains how polarity affects today's youth.

Flower Essences

Flower essences were originally discovered by a medical doctor from England, Dr. Edward Bach. Dr. Bach (pronounced Batch) sensed that the dew on flowers had special healing properties and began to experiment with his patients. Because it was impractical and difficult to collect water from blooms, he picked flowers and let them soak in a crystal bowl in the sunlight to extract the healing properties; this extraction he called the mother tincture. Before use it was further diluted. Unlike homeopathy, these remedies cure problems with healthful, positive energy; homeopathy uses a diluted toxic substance to provide a cure.

Dr. Bach believed the healings occurred because the procedure used all of the elements: The earth to nurture the plant, the air from which it feeds, the sun or fire to enable it to impart its power, and water to collect and be enriched with its beneficent magnetic healing.5

These remedies work on the emotional state which might actually cause or at least contribute largely to the physical illness or issue. For example, many flower essence practitioners believe that if people are given larch, it will help them improve their feelings of self-esteem. Resentment may be associated with cancer, according to Louise Hay in *You Can Heal Your Life*. Therefore, adding willow flower essence or a flower essence combination including willow would be appropriate support for someone with cancer. Some manufacturers make combinations with names specific to their purpose, for example, Resolve Anger, Safe Boundaries, Calm Child, and Rescue Remedy.

Here are Bach's thirty-eight essences and their indications:

- Agrimony – mental torture behind a cheerful face
- Aspen – fear of unknown things
- Beech – intolerance
- Centaury – inability to say, No
- Cerato – lack of trust in one's own decisions
- Cherry Plum – fear of the mind giving way
- Chestnut Bud (made with horse chestnut buds) – failure to learn from mistakes
- Chicory – selfish, possessive love
- Clematis – dreaming of the future without working in the present
- Crab Apple – cleansing remedy, also for self-hatred
- Elm – overwhelmed by responsibility
- Gentian – discouragement after a setback
- Gorse – hopelessness and despair
- Heather – self-centeredness and self-concern
- Holly – hatred, envy and jealousy
- Honeysuckle – living in the past
- Hornbeam – procrastination, tiredness at the thought of doing something
- Impatiens – impatience
- Larch – lack of confidence and self-esteem
- Mimulus – fear of known things
- Mustard – deep gloom for no reason
- Oak – the plodder who keeps going past the point of exhaustion
- Olive – exhaustion following mental or physical effort
- Pine – guilt
- Red Chestnut (a type of horse chestnut) – over-concern for the welfare of loved ones
- Rock Rose – terror and fright
- Rock Water – self-denial, rigidity and self-repression
- Scleranthus – inability to choose between alternatives

- Star of Bethlehem – shock
- Sweet Chestnut – Extreme mental anguish, when everything has been tried, and there is no light left
- Vervain – over-enthusiasm
- Vine – dominance and inflexibility
- Walnut – protection from change and unwanted influences
- Water Violet – pride and aloofness
- White Chestnut (made with horse chestnut blossoms) – unwanted thoughts and mental arguments
- Wild Oat – uncertainty over one's direction in life
- Wild Rose – drifting, resignation, apathy
- Willow – self-pity and resentment. 6

Homeopathy

Both homeopathy and flower essence therapies go against conventional medical wisdom, and according to the study of chemistry and pharmacology, should not be effective. Throughout the countries of the world, many M.D.'s are also classical homeopaths, although having an M.D. is not a requirement. Homeopathy was discovered in the 18th century by Dr. Samuel Hahnemann, a German physician, when he found that a substance that caused symptoms similar to a disease might cure it. As with essences, he so diluted the materials that they were not toxic, but they provided the impetus to a cure. These also work on emotional and physical issues of a patient. Homeopathy is a complex study, and in certain countries such as Argentina, only a licensed M.D. can administer homeopathic remedies, yet science in general discounts any effect other than placebo. Herbalists and naturopaths often use mild homeopathic remedies. Some of the most effective ones are for teething babies (calcium phosphate and chamomilla), soreness and pain (arnica), and fever blisters (Borax, Antimonium Crudum, Baptisia Tinctoria 3X HPUS Natrum Muriaticum). Hylands has a line of remedies for everything a family needs. Although many dispute their effectiveness, they are apparently very safe and widely used throughout the world.

Reiki. Healing Touch. Touch for Health. The Reconnection. The Divine Matrix

The general public's interest in energy healing sky rocketed at the turn of the 21st century; in fact, many hospitals are now allowing nurses and Reiki healers to provide healing energy to people undergoing surgical procedures. While each of these energy methods has distinctive rituals, practices, etc., they all work on the principle that we can use divine energy by focusing it or channeling it with intention, with the use of symbols or without. Sometimes the results astound the client, and other times they may barely perceive any change.

Many times, a person will receive a healing and afterwards say something like, 'That was nice, but I didn't feel a thing'. Later on, however, people have been known to see dramatic changes in their situations. Apparently, as Eric Pearle of The Reconnection says, God decides upon the healing. We are just the instrument or the tool. 7 The proper healing for that person at that time always occurs. My first experience with the results of Reiki happened when I sprained my ankle badly while walking around a fall festival in a large downtown area over a mile from my home. Jayson, a Reiki master, offered to treat me with Reiki. Not even knowing what Reiki was, I agreed to anything that might help take away the pain. He held my ankle for ten minutes, until he felt the heat go away. Immediately, I was able to walk around the rest of the festival and all of the way home. The next day, I had some soreness, but no real pain.

That experience convinced me that I needed to be attuned to Reiki. Later that year, after my attunement (ritualistic introduction) to Reiki, I entered a group healing about 10 minutes after the three other Reiki practitioners had begun a healing on Sherry, a woman with hepatitis C. She was lying on the massage table, and the others were at her head, her feet, and her side. For the next thirty minutes or so, I saw tiny orange triangles bouncing off of Sherry's abdomen. When the healing was complete, I asked the others if they had seen the orange figures or if they knew what it meant. Jayson seemed surprised at my question, walked across the room, picked up a sheet of paper with an orange triangle printed on it, and announced that before I had come, they had decided to do pyramid healing on Sherry. I had SEEN the pyramids focused on the problem area.

William Lee Rand has the most comprehensive website I have seen on energy healing, and although the focus is on Reiki, it applies to all types of healings: www.reiki.org. The following passage and more information can be found on the reiki.org web site:

How Does Reiki Work?

We are alive because life force is flowing through us. Life force flows within the physical body through pathways called chakras, meridians and nadis. It also flows around us in a field of energy called the aura. Life force nourishes the organs and cells of the body, supporting them in their vital functions. When this flow of life force is disrupted, it causes diminished function in one or more of the organs and tissues of the physical body

The life force is responsive to thoughts and feelings. It becomes disrupted when we accept, either consciously or unconsciously, negative thoughts or feelings about ourselves. These negative thoughts and feelings attach themselves to the energy field and cause a disruption in the flow of life force. This diminishes the vital function of the organs and cells of the physical body.

Reiki heals by flowing through the affected parts of the energy field and charging them with positive energy. It raises the vibratory level of the energy field in and around the physical body where the negative thoughts and feelings are attached. This causes the negative energy to break apart and fall away. In so doing, Reiki clears, straightens and heals the energy pathways, thus allowing the life force to flow in a healthy and natural way.

HEALING TOUCH

Healing Touch is widely used by nurses and other healers. There is now an insurance code for healing work performed by a certified healing touch practitioner. Healing Touch is a relaxing, nurturing energy therapy. Gentle touch assists in balancing your physical, mental, emotional, and spiritual well-being. Healing Touch works with the energy field to support your natural ability to heal. It is safe for all ages and works in harmony with standard medical care (healingtouch.com).

HOW CAN HEALING TOUCH BENEFIT YOU?

- Reducing stress
- Calming anxiety, depression
- Decreasing pain
- Strengthening the immune system
- Enhancing recovery from surgery
- Complementing care for neck and back problems
- Deepening spiritual connection
- Supporting cancer care
- Creating a sense of well-being
- Easing acute and chronic conditions

Obviously, from the above descriptions, we have nothing to fear from Reiki and healing touch or any of the other wonderful modalities of healing...and everything to gain. I encourage all people to find a healer that they can trust and one with whom they are comfortable in order to experience energy work and its many benefits.

Another well-established school of healing is the Barbara Brennan School of Energy. Brennan is a former NASA physicist and an author of several books on energy work, including the bestselling *Hands of Light and Light Emerging*. Her curriculum involves several years of study in a very intense program where students must meet five times a year with her to practice and evolve as healers.

I had a wonderful experience with a graduate of this school. Having been told by Dr. Danielle LoRito of Italy that I had a hidden anger that must be resolved, I turned to Marianne, a Brennan energy graduate, for help. Marianne cleared eight layers of energy around my liver area. For one month afterwards, yellow flakes (yellow is the color of the liver area chakra and the color of bile) came from under the fingernails on my right hand only. The liver is on the right side of the body. The right side is also the father; my father abandoned the family when I was only two years old. The healing definitely occurred, and the wound was closed.

Reflexology

Reflexology is an ancient, but newly rediscovered art which uses the feet, the hands and the ears to reach reflex points deep within the body. Basically, Dr. William Fitzgerald introduced these concepts to the West almost 100 years ago. Eunice Ingham further refined his zone therapy into

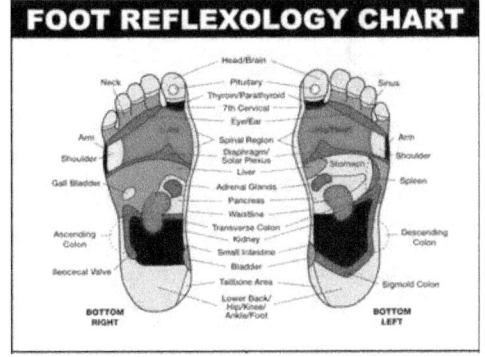

what is now known as Reflexology. By massaging certain zones on the feet, the reflexologist can evoke a healing in different organs and tissues of the body by bringing the body back into balance. Not only does reflexology feel great (who doesn't like a deep foot rub?), it can help a person sleep better, ease arthritis pain and back pain, and help many other health issues. Essential oils applied to specific areas or colored lights applied to the reflex points on the foot or the ear will improve conditions in the body.

Essential oils require a book unto themselves, and I highly recommend reading *Reference Guide for Essential Oils* by Connie and Alan Higley.

There are reflex points on the teeth as each tooth lies along a meridian. I once heard a great story from a breast cancer survivor who had been going to a holistic dentist to have her mercury removed. During the process, she had to have a tooth removed; when they pulled it, she broke down in tears and felt a huge release. The dentist showed her this tooth chart and said that he had just pulled her breast tooth!

Meridian Tooth Chart

Joints	Right Shoulder, elbow, hand (ulnar), S.I. joint, foot, toes	Right: TMJ, anterior hip/knee, medial ankle	Right: Shoulder-elbow-hand (radial), foot, big toe	Right: Posterior knee, hip, lateral ankle	Right: Posterior knee, sacro-coccygeal joint, posterior ankle	Left: Posterior knee, sacro-coccygeal joint, posterior ankle	Left: Posterior knee, hip, lateral ankle	Left: Shoulder-elbow-hand (radial), foot, big toe	Left: TMJ, anterior hip/knee, medial ankle	Left: Shoulder-elbow-hand (ulnar), S.I joint, foot, toes
Mammary Glands		R i g h t B r e a s t							L e f t B r e a s t	
Endocrine Glands	Anterior pituitary	Parathyroid	Thyroid	Thymus	Posterior pituitary	Intermediate lobe of pituitary	Pineal	Pineal	Intermediate lobe of pituitary	Posterior pituitary	Thymus	Thyroid	Parathyroid	Anterior pituitary
Organs	Right heart, right duodenum, terminal ileum	Pancreas, right side of stomach, esophagus	Right lung, right side of large intestine	Right side of liver, gall bladder, right side of biliary ducts	Right kidney, bladder, uterus, prostate, rectum, anus	Left kidney, bladder, uterus, prostate, rectum, anus	Left side of liver, biliary ducts	Left lung, left side of large intestine	Spleen, left side of stomach, esophagus	Left heart, left side of duodenum, jejunum, ileum
Teeth Pictured	Retromolar													Retromolar
Names of Teeth	Right upper 3rd molar (wisdom)	Right upper 2nd molar	Right upper 1st molar	Right upper 2nd bicuspid (pre-molar)	Right upper 1st bicuspid (pre-molar)	Right upper canine (cuspid)	Right upper lateral incisor	Right upper central incisor	Left upper central incisor	Left upper lateral incisor	Left upper canine (cuspid)	Left upper 1st bicuspid (pre-molar)	Left upper 2nd bicuspid (pre-molar)	Left upper 1st molar	Left upper 2nd molar	Left upper 3rd molar (wisdom)
American Nomenclature	1	2	3	4	5	6	7	8	9	10	11	12	13	14	15	16
	32	31	30	29	28	27	26	25	24	23	22	21	20	19	18	17
Names of Teeth	Right lower 3rd molar (wisdom)	Right lower 2nd molar	Right lower 1st molar	Right lower 2nd bicuspid (pre-molar)	Right lower 1st bicuspid (pre-molar)	Right lower canine (cuspid)	Right lower lateral incisor	Right lower central incisor	Left lower central incisor	Left lower lateral incisor	Left lower canine (cuspid)	Left lower 1st bicuspid (pre-molar)	Left lower 2nd bicuspid (pre-molar)	Left lower 1st molar	Left lower 2nd molar	Left lower 3rd molar (wisdom)
Teeth Pictured	Retromolar													Retromolar
Organs	Right heart, terminal ileum, duodenum	Pancreas, right side of stomach, pylorus, esophagus	Right lung, right side of large intestine	Right side of liver, gall bladder, right side of biliary ducts	Right kidney, bladder, uterus, prostate, rectum, anus	Left kidney, bladder, uterus, prostate, rectum, anus	Left side of liver, biliary ducts	Left lung, left side of large intestine	Spleen, left side of stomach, esophagus	Left heart, left side of duodenum, jejunum, ileum
Endocrine Glands				Ovaries,	testicles	Adrenals	Adrenals	Ovaries,	testicles				
Mammary glands		R i g h t B r e a s t							L e f t B r e a s t	
Joints	Right Shoulder, elbow, hand (ulnar), S.I joint, foot, toes	Right: TMJ, anterior hip/knee, medial ankle	Right: Shoulder-elbow-hand (radial), foot, big toe	Right: Posterior knee, hip, lateral ankle	Right: Posterior knee, sacro-coccygeal joint, posterior ankle	Left: Posterior knee, sacro-coccygeal joint, posterior ankle	Left: Posterior knee, hip, lateral ankle	Left: Shoulder-elbow-hand (radial), foot, big toe	Left: TMJ, anterior hip/knee, medial ankle	Left: Shoulder-elbow-hand (ulnar), S.I joint, foot, toes

BioAcoustics

BioAcoustics is a field of research documenting the ability of sound to support the human body's ability to diagnose and heal itself.

Sharry Edwards, guided by her unique abilities to hear sounds beyond the normal human spectrum and her ability to influence human physiology with the sounds of her voice, began developing the techniques of human BioAcoustics in 1982. Today, as the executive director of Sound Health Alternatives International, Inc. of Albany, Ohio, a non-profit research center, Sharry Edwards continues her research and trains and certifies health care practitioners in the use of healing sound techniques.[31]

The process involves two steps: voice spectral analysis (Vocal Profiling) and the presentation of low-frequency sound.

A healthy body produces a full spectrum of harmonious frequencies. So, a BioAcoustic research associate (BARA) first records and analyzes sounds produced in normal speech; then, based on a voice's pattern of both deficient and/or over-abundant frequencies, selects a series of sounds to aid the body in bringing itself back into harmony. These low-frequency analog sound sets may be delivered by either earphones or a speaker.

The types of energy work above are but a sampling of the major categories of healing energy being practiced. If you haven't experienced the benefits of these energies, now would be a very good time to get started. One of the wonderful aspects of it all is that each time you offer God's healing energy to someone else, you receive a wonderful healing treatment yourself.

---

[31] Sound Health Alternatives maintains the website nutrasounds.com.

Challenges for Week Five

☐ Look for one of these alternative practitioners in your area. If you don't connect completely with the first person you try, try someone else. Visit an iridologist, sclerologist, or BioAcoustic practitioner.

☐ Experience an energy healing – Reiki, Healing Touch, Barbara Brennan, The Reconnection. Be patient waiting for the results; they might be subtle but real.

☐ Study the tooth chart and reflexology charts.

☐ Have you or do you have a tooth that is bothering you? Where is it on the reflex chart? Try some "Tooth Tonic" and clean with baking soda and food grade peroxide.

☐ Study the chakras to learn where you need balance. Wear the colors you need to come into balance; for example, blue for clear communication, red for grounding, and purple for enlightenment.

Week Six: Deep Tissue and Colon Cleansing

It is important to remember that we can't keep our bodies clean without cleaning up our exterior living environment. In this chapter, we will take steps to cleanse inside our bodies:

- ☐ Practice an alkaline lifestyle

- ☐ Consider limited use of the microwave, x-rays, and the cell phone. Use EMF protection such as sacred geometry or protective diodes.

- ☐ Eat more raw, cleansing vegetables and fruits.

- ☐ Fast one day a month or one day a week.

- ☐ Follow the Master Cleanse Lemon Diet for 1-10 days.

- ☐ Do a deep tissue and colon cleanse at least once a year.

- ☐ Flush the kidneys using kidney herbs and pure, alkaline water before you stir up toxins in the bowel.

- ☐ Practice deep breathing to saturate the tissues with oxygen and increase pH levels.

- ☐ Watch out because cleansing the body might lead to cleaning out the attic, the garage, and the kitchen junk drawer, too.

Cleansing

"The uncleanness within is greater than the uncleanness without. And he who cleanses himself without, but within remains unclean, is like a tomb that outward is painted fair, but is within full of all manner of horrible uncleannesses and abominations."
- Essene Gospel of Jesus

Cleansing, which has been practiced for thousands of years, was written about as early as the Essene Gospels of Jesus. Today, cleansing is a popular concept promoted by naturopaths and many herbalists and advertised on television infomercials at all hours of the day and night. All of the hype makes us wonder whether cleansing is a valid concern. But today's lifestyles make removing toxic build up from the lining of the intestines more important than ever. A good cleanse builds and cleans the blood, kidneys, liver, and gallbladder and relieves stress on the whole body. Animals know to clean themselves by eating certain grasses to promote vomiting or diarrhea. And, because we care about our pets, we humans worm them once a year to help them remove their load of undesirable parasites. HELLO! What about us? Don't we deserve to be treated as well as our animals?

From our food, air, and water supplies and exposure to chemicals through medicines, vaccines, exhaust fumes, carpet cleaners, preservatives, food – you name it – we are all bombarded with foreign substances our organic bodies can't cope with. The body tucks them away in areas such as the lining of the digestive tract, under the skin in the form of cellulite, and as plaque in our arteries. As discussed earlier, to top it off, we are eating and drinking much more sugar and over- processed foods than ever before. Then we use sedatives and stimulants to get through the day and artificial sweeteners, the icing on the cake of illness, to avoid more sugar. I'll never forget a demonstration by Dr. Bernard Jensen, one I have repeated many times. He put an aspirin, but any pill will do, in a spoon over a candle flame. We watched as the white, round pill turned into a black, tarry soup of asphalt-looking material. This black goop indicates what pills do inside the body... turn into plaque buildup. This black tarry material can get pulled out of the body during a colon cleanse.

How clean are you inside? Could you have a toxic body? On the outside, we scrub our bodies, our teeth and our hair every day in this country, but unless our colon "backs up" or "acts up," we tend to ignore internal scrubbing. Perhaps we would be wise to look there before we manifest these health issues. Just take a look at the short list of symptoms relating to poor colon health:

- IBS
- Parasites
- Gas
- Fatigue
- Stomach cramps
- Toxic uterus
- Pain
- Prostate problems
- Body odor
- Allergies
- Eczema
- Congestion

People who have a pattern of constipation sometimes rely on harsh laxatives (which won't continue to work forever), enemas and suppositories. In fact, many get to the point of relying totally on outside means to produce bowel movements because the peristalsis is barely working, or the balance of bacteria is off. Loose bowels are still an imbalance in the body, another form of constipation, as the body isn't getting the absorption it needs from the diet.

Dr. Linda Berry, a chiropractor and clinical nutritionist, summarizes the symptoms of self-poisoning:

- Bad breath and foul-smelling gas and stools
- Constipation, diarrhea, sluggish elimination
- Frequent congestion, colds, viruses
- Flatulence or gas and frequent intestinal disorders
- Frequent headaches for no apparent reason
- Migrating aches and pains
- Intolerance to fatty foods
- Low energy; loss of vitality for no apparent reason
- Lower back pain
- Lowered resistance to infections
- Needing to sleep a long time
- Pain in the liver or gall bladder
- Premenstrual syndrome (PMS), breast soreness, vaginal infections
- Skin problems, rashes, boils, pimples, acne[32]

If you have serious health problems, seek the attention of a competent health care provider, but anyone who has been on the Standard American Diet (SAD Diet) for more than two years would benefit from cleansing.[33]

Assuming that almost everyone has or has had some of the above symptoms, can we deduce that everyone needs a cleanse. Do you? Take the quiz below to see whether or not you need a detox cleanse.

☐ Do you have one or fewer bowel movements each day?

☐ Are you feeling sluggish or tired?

☐ Do you have dry skin, psoriasis or eczema?

☐ Do you gain weight without overeating?

---

[32] Berry, Linda, Dr. *Internal Cleansing.* www.drlindaberry.com/interclean.php. Accessed May 5, 2007.
[33] Dr Natura. *Are You Clean Inside?* www.drnatura.com. Accessed March, 2005.

- ☐ Do you have a lot of food and chemical sensitivities?

- ☐ Does smoke make you feel sick?

- ☐ Are your hair or nails weak or do they break off easily?

- ☐ Do you feel bloated or do you have excess gas?

- ☐ Do you experience body odor or bad breath?

- ☐ Do you have sinus problems, colds, or other congestion often?

- ☐ Do you have mood swings or do you feel stressed?

So, what are the benefits of colon and deep tissue cleansing for you? It is no miracle cure, but . . .

- • If you need to lose weight, a cleanse will be a great start!
- • If you want to quit smoking, a cleanse will help you lose your dependence on nicotine.
- • If you want more energy, a cleanse will help restore vitality.
- • If you just want to purify your body and spirit, a cleanse brings clarity and purity.
- • If you need to alkalize, the most cleansing diet is plant-based and raw, so add more smoothies and salads to your diet.

Is it possible that cleansing could help to prevent illness and improve emotional well-being? Is it also possible that cleaning the blood, kidneys, liver, and colon would help not only digestion, but also relieve us of allergies and minimize the effects of aging? Of course it is possible. Anyone who has been on a lengthy fast or a month-long cleansing program can attest to the heightened feelings of spiritual connectedness. The AT-ONE-MENT with God and all other beings naturally occurs when we quit bombarding our system with JUNK and begin nourishing our being with wholesome food and fresh vegetable and fruit juices.

Twenty years ago, my husband and I did our first cleanse together based upon Dr. Richard Anderson's book, Cleanse and Purify Thyself. We went all out:

daily colonics, tons of water and fresh-squeezed juices, no meats or starches. All the while, we were cooking nightly for our three children, preparing school lunches and doing everything else that goes along with running a household, yet after a couple of days, we had no DESIRE to eat "normal foods." We were not working for that month, so we had time at home (free time is important to devoting oneself to cleansing, especially while doing colonics). After the first ten to fourteen days, we lost all interest in food and had to force ourselves to drink juices; our heightened spirituality both consumed and thrilled us. Life became a meditation (of course, it always was; we had just been too busy to see it).

Since that time, the effects of that cleanse have stayed with us, encouraging us to participate in further cleanse programs and helping us to support others in their cleansing efforts. Cleansing brought about such positive changes in my body that internal detoxification became a passionate part of my life, as well as a main component in my nutritional practice. Proper bowel function entails having 2 to 3 normal (not loose) bowel movements per day, and many people need to cleanse and cleanse again in order to become that regular. Some will never achieve the goal of eliminating after each meal, but everyone can improve. People who have a bowel movement once a week (yes, there are many) MUST move their bowels more often. When we don't eliminate our waste, toxins back up and can cause autointoxication or self- poisoning. Blood capillaries lining the bowel wall begin to absorb these toxins into the bloodstream, consequently polluting all of our organs and cells. Cleansing will help to kill parasites, limit yeast problems, increase absorption, and enable the body to heal itself.

Diet is an important part of the cleansing process, but changing the diet is not imperative to receiving some benefits from the program. I have seen "cleansers" receive wonderful improvements in their health even without giving up meat and coffee; while they might not receive the full benefits, the herbs, clays, fibers, etc. pull toxins from the body even while a person is putting other toxic substances in. Meat, most grains, refined carbohydrates and sugars steal electrolytes from the body.

Mucoid plaque forms along the digestive tract to protect the body from super acidic bile which becomes more and more acid in the absence of enough electrolytes. This plaque interferes with assimilation of nutrients and digestion; toxins aren't properly eliminated and the body accumulates undesirable micro-organisms, developing yeasts, bacteria, viruses and parasites that rob the body of nutrients and contribute to acid waste in

When the bowel is toxic, the blood picks up the toxins and takes them to the liver, eventually polluting the entire body and making it difficult to stay healthy or overcome illness (*Arise and Shine*). According to Dr. Bernard Jensen, "Every tissue in the body is fed by the bloodstream, which is supplied by the bowel. When the bowel is dirty, the blood is dirty and so are the organs and tissues. It is the bowel that must be cared for first."[34]

While we care for the bowel, we also are relieving stress on our other filtration systems: the liver, lungs, kidneys, skin and lymphatic drainage systems. When any one of these "helper" systems is backed up, it adversely affects all of the others. Back ache is often related to a toxic colon, but isn't it also connected to the kidneys as well? And isn't it true that skin eruptions reflect a toxic body that isn't eliminating properly, so the skin, a secondary organ of elimination, is assisting the colon and the liver by pushing toxins out? And isn't it strange that the current treatment for chronic acne is low-dose antibiotics – just kill everything, good, bad and whatever. A person can't get off of the antibiotics because the good bacteria are gone, too!

An important part of some cleansing programs includes some kind of clay to alkalize and draw toxins through the intestinal wall. Bentonite clay is somewhat

---

[34] Jensen, Bernard, Dr. *Tissue Cleaning Through Bowel Management.* New York: Avery Press, 1999..

different from the other types of clay because when water is added to Bentonite, the molecular structure changes and an electrical charge is produced. The clay attracts toxins into the mixture which bind to the clay because of the electric charge. The largest deposits of this volcanic ash clay are found in Wyoming and Montana. It is sun dried for use in baths and facials.

The body has various pathways which can eliminate waste and toxins: the kidneys, the bowels, the lungs, and our largest secondary organ of elimination – the skin. Remember that the kidneys have to filter out toxins like heavy metals and mineral build up. The kidney is particularly sensitive and performs much better when it is clean and functioning at a high level. A kidney produces and cleans up to a gallon of urine every day! Remember that in Week One we began skin brushing before showering; this practice is cleansing in that it exfoliates the skin and allows toxins to escape.

In naturopathy, we use the expression, "Never stop a flow." This means to allow toxins, mucus, and infections to leave the body. When you have a runny nose, for goodness sakes don't take anything to stop it. This is your body's way of saying, "Help. I need to get rid of this stuff!" The same is true of the colon. When people come into my office and say that they have a bowel movement every 3 – 7 days, it is past time to get things moving. Imagine the cesspool their uterus is living in or skin eruptions, headaches, menstrual problems… the list goes on. Books on cleansing abound, and in addition to Dr. Anderson's Arise and Shine, is Dr. Bernard Jensen's Tissue Cleansing Through Bowel Management. While there are many websites dedicated to this topic, it is best to find a health practitioner who specializes in deep tissue and bowel cleansing to direct your process and assist you in having a positive experience.

The Master Cleanse

Dr. Stanley Burroughs researched cleansing and published a book on the now popular "Master Cleanse."[35] This liquid diet has been called the Lemonade Diet as well. Many like to include it as an integral part of any cleansing program or, as Dr. Burroughs claims, the lemon mixture supplies all of the nutrition needed and deep cleans even for diabetics. Below are two versions of his recipe:

Master Cleanser Morning Drink (One serving)

2 cups water
1/2 or 1 squeezed lemon
1 – 2 T. Organic Grade B Maple Syrup
Dash cayenne pepper
Mix together and drink in the morning before drinking anything else.

People have reported clearer skin, better bowel movements, more energy, etc. Some people have fasted using just this drink with no solid food with a good effect on weight and health. The below recipe makes 60 oz of "lemonade," enough for 6 to 10 oz glasses.

One Half Gallon of Master Cleanse

64 oz water
12 tablespoons Organic Grade B Maple Syrup
12 tablespoons freshly squeezed lemon juice (or 2 tbsp. per glass) a little over half a teaspoon of cayenne pepper (or 1/10 tsp. per glass) or to taste .4

Use less maple syrup if it is too sweet and think about this: participants in this program have had bowel movements 10 days into this cleanse, with no solid food!

---

[35] Borroughs, Stanley. Master Cleanse Secrets. www.mastercleansesecrets.com/book. Accessed May 2005.

Adjuncts to Cleansing

Some of the latest thoughts on acid reflux are that people's systems are so backed up that food can't completely leave the stomach, so the stomach produces more and more acid, trying to digest the small amount of food remaining in the stomach– the problem is that it has nowhere to go due to constipation or incomplete elimination. Many types of cleanses will help this problem, but important adjuncts to cleansing include the liver-gallbladder cleanse, castor oil pack, and salt water or coffee enemas. Nothing is as important as green vegetable smoothies and other blended drinks.

Liver-Gallbladder Cleanse

Save the gallbladder! Try the liver-gallbladder cleanse; recipes vary but it involves drinking olive oil and fresh lemon or grapefruit juice at night before bed time. Dr. Hulda Clark recommends using Epsom Salts to speed elimination and to force the bile ducts open, but it seems to work very well without that harsh purgative. Take some cascara sagrada or drink an herbal laxative tea if you need help with elimination. If you do this while going through a cleansing program, you won't need a thing to move the bowels. You may need to perform the treatment several times before you get the desired result, but almost everyone feels better right away. Usually, folks pass a lot of little green balls that Hulda Clark, in her excellent book *The Cure For All Diseases*, assures us are forming gall stones. One of my clients took them to a local lab to have them analyzed; the report confirmed that they were unknown "inorganic matter." Who knows? Maybe they are those crayons we ate in first grade or just the paraffin from the Snickers we ate in college. Please consult Dr. Clark's work for her full view of cleansing and a logical order to conduct cleansing programs for parasites, the kidneys, the liver, the bowel, and the blood.

Castor Oil Pack

Castor oil is the only oil known to contain ricinoleic acid, an unusual unsaturated fatty acid that has amazing healing properties. It has been shown to boost the immune system and inhibit viruses, molds, and yeasts. It builds the immune system as it increases production of lymphocytes in the body. Dr. David Williams says it was called the Palma Christe "because the shape of the plant's leaves was thought to resemble the palm of Christ." He goes on to say, "As familiar as I am with the healing power of this plant, the name may be very accurate."

To do a castor oil pack on the abdomen, soak a flannel cloth with castor oil, put it over the abdomen and cover with plastic wrap or a plastic bag. Put the heating pad on for an hour or more and get instant relief from reflux and soothing aid for the liver and gallbladder.[36]

Cleansing Through Breath

Increasing oxygen to the cells through deep breathing is logical – more oxygen deeper into the lungs increases health at the cellular level. Take a deep breath and feel your body relax. In as little as five minutes a day, we can breathe our way to good health; of course, in this case more is better. Yoga, QiGong, and Tai Chi, as well as many aerobic activities, utilize the breath as a tool to increase stamina and concentration. With enough oxygen to the cells, the body repairs itself adequately. An intensive breathwork session such as conscious connected breathing not only helps participants move into an altered state and release stored suppression, but can also raise the pH and promote an alkalizing, cleansing condition.

---

[36] Borroughs, Stanley. *Master Cleanse Secrets*. www.mastercleansesecrets.com/book. Accessed May 2005.

One of my clients began checking her pH before and after a breath session. At the beginning of each session, her pH registered between 5 and 6, very low, reflecting her ill health; at the end, after an hour of intensive breathing, her pH shot up to 8 or even 8 1/2. While I don't know of any clinical trials that have been done, this one case shows some of the power of breathing, something we do every minute to survive this brief lifetime. To get this level of increase in pH might require intensive work or a yoga class at least, but if a person just begins to watch the breath and to breathe deeply into the abdomen – deep belly breaths as the yogis say – he or she will begin to see the results in oxygen to the cells and better energy.

Cleansing Tips

Remind yourself about what we read earlier about pH (alkalinity) and diet. Check your pH; if your saliva and urine are testing below 7 (neutral), your electrolyte and alkaline reserves may too acidic for cleansing.

Consider drinking kidney/and/or parsley tea before and during cleansing. To make parsley tea, simmer 1 bunch parsley for 20 minutes in 1 quart of water with a lid on the pot. Strain and drink 2 cups per day. If you have a history of kidney or bladder issues, be sure to take additional herbal kidney support such as Dr. Christopher or Blue Boy Herb Kidney Formula and drink about a gallon of alkaline water per day.

A cleanse doesn't require supplements, but certainly taking some will make it more efficient and effective. While cleansing (not fasting) we should provide certain nutrients that will energize and nourish the body during the cleansing process. Drink vegetable juices and soups, drink alkaline water and green powder or juice drinks to promote alkalinity and an environment conducive to healing. Cleansing program ideas and references follow this list.

During a cleanse, it is normal to have reactions as the blood stream collects toxins and gets "worse" before it gets better. Cleansing reactions should be brief, generally, although recently Dr. Robert Young explained in his newsletter why so many people get "influenza" during the holidays. ITS NOT THE FLU! It is the body's reaction to an acidic lifestyle – chips and dips, cheese balls and crackers, lots of wine, pie and eggnog. If what he says is true, keeping alkaline whether cleansing or not must be pretty important.[37]

Cleansing and Purifying: The Secret to Good Health

Over the last twenty years, we have introduced hundreds of people to the protocols and products that help the body cleanse out impurities. At times, the results have been outstanding and amazing. Cleansing not only empties the body of toxic waste; it also releases toxic emotions along with the waste. People report feeling better physically and emotionally – extra pounds, skin irritations, depression – these things and more are known to melt away while following a cleansing diet.

Congratulations to you for taking the first step to investigate this process and to see if it is for you. I admire you for being willing to get started on your own self-healing program. While you proceed, remember to think good thoughts and to be open to the positive changes occurring in your body and spirit. I pray that you will have the result you are hoping for and that you will find the strength to follow through with your new life program.

The most critical key to vibrant health is maintaining proper elimination of toxins from the body, while eating living foods that allow the body to heal and rebuild itself. Although at first it may seem complicated to make these changes,

---

[37] Young, Robert. Holiday Season Influenza or 'I Ate Too Much'

once you become accustomed to the program and how good you feel while doing it, it becomes exciting and simple.

So, What's Your Problem?

Are you constipated? Do you have diarrhea? How about gas, bloating, indigestion, headaches, body aches, bad breath, allergies, skin rashes, asthma, irritable bowel, memory loss, chronic fatigue, back aches, fibromyalgia, insomnia, infertility, weight problems, candida overgrowth, immune function disorders, arthritis, or frequent illnesses? These problems and others can be symptoms of auto-intoxication. When the body can no longer deal with unhealthy habits, it begins to exhibit symptoms such as those listed above. If these problems are not dealt with in a timely manner, they can lead to more serious health issues in the days and years ahead. Find out how you can become active in offsetting any of these problems in a healthy, body- friendly way through an individualized cleansing program.

Understanding the Cleansing: What to Eat

Meat, sugar, and many grains are acid-forming foods that rob you of important electrolytes, causing the bile to become more and more acid. A more acid bile leads to plaque forming along the intestinal tract, inhibiting digestion and assimilation of nutrients. Meanwhile, the toxicity in the bowel is assimilated into the blood stream and taken back to the liver. From here, the entire body is affected, and the body loses its ability to heal. At this point, people gain weight, form cellulite, have headaches... as they head toward more serious disorders. This is where many people find themselves when they decide to try cleansing to restore their health.

While cleansing it is best to eat alkaline, vegetarian, and primarily raw. Sprouted and soaked grains and nuts and seeds are great, but limit them while cleansing as they slow down the process. Millet and quinoa, though more alkaline-forming grains, should only be eaten to compliment your vegetables.

Breakfast might consist of your lemon water (a master cleanse), followed by fresh fruit. Do not mix citrus or melons with other fruits. A green smoothie is great at this time, and if you add extra virgin coconut oil and flax seeds, it will be filling enough to sustain you through the morning. Another good smoothie while cleansing is raw almond milk with vanilla and coconut oil. Throw in some raw coconut for sweetness. Lunch should be a good vegetable soup or broth or some raw or steamed vegetables with seeds or nuts (soaked first). Kitcheree (see recipe) is good at this time. Salads or roasted vegetables with herbs are also delicious

Dinner should be as many vegetables as you like. The snack ideas in Week Three will help you make the transition to a more alkaline diet. Limit yourself to organic cold-pressed organic olive, coconut, and flax oils. Try to eat 80% raw. If you have sugar or yeast problems, stick to vegetables and vegetable juices.

What to Expect

You will feel better most of the time, and when the cleanse is going good, you will feel great! There are many different reactions to cleansing, but most people will expect something like the following:

A healthy person might have 3 or 4 bowel movements per day; one first thing in the morning and one after each meal. People that have a constipative pattern will be surprised to find that they can increase their bowel movements to this point with the use of cleansing herbs and an alkaline diet.

If you are not having an increase in bowel movements, you should increase the amount of water and master cleanser and consider more raw veggies and smoothies. Don't be worried. A highly-constipated person may take 3 – 5 times the amount of laxative herbs or minerals such as Cascara Sagrada or magnesium to cleanse the bowels. Never stay constipated. Take a plain or salt water enema to relieve the toxins if necessary.

If while cleansing, the bowels are too loose, take less of the cleansing product. If instructions tell you to take them three times a day, go down to two times, etc.

As mucoid plaque is breaking down, it may show up in the stools as shiny black, grey, green, orange leathery stripes of even ropes. It often does not immediately fall apart in the water.

Cleansing Reactions

Diarrhea, constipation, headaches, nausea, fatigue, even night sweats may all be signs that the body is pulling out toxins faster than the kidneys and bowels can eliminate them. Relief might come from an enema or colonic and more alkaline water or water with lemon and cayenne.

A coffee enema (organic, unroasted coffee with purified water only) will really stimulate the liver to work better and has been used in alternative cancer treatments. Colonics are another option and are a good adjunct to speeding up the cleansing process. Some cleansing reactions are solved by drinking enough pure water – about 1 oz. per pound of body weight while cleansing.

Will I Get Enough Protein?

More people suffer from too much protein in their diet already (the SAD – Standard American Diet), but the myth that we all lack protein lives on. Meat eaters may assimilate less protein than vegetable eaters because of poor liver and digestive function. Fruits and vegetables contain more protein than most people realize. Comprehensive studies done on protein and its harmful effects in the body are discussed in Dr. Campbell's *The China Study*, a must read for those worrying about cancer in modern society. See the acid/alkaline chart for more information for getting alkaline.

Cleansing does not take the place of medical attention, and anyone under a doctor's care and beginning a cleansing program should advise their physician at the onset of the program.

Don't forget about other needs for cleansing such as cell phones, x-rays, and microwaves. People react to any mention of this danger as if it were a bizarre suggestion that only a fanatic would be concerned with; however, testing has shown this to be a real danger.

A rating for all cell phones is called the SAR rating (Specific Absorption Rating) or how much radiation your brain is absorbing. Wireless home phones are almost just as dangerous, apparently, and it is wise to limit the time you spend on the phone to one or two minutes at most. Microwave dangers have been discussed for many years, and research concludes that they emit strong fields of radiation. So, if you use a cell or portable phone, if you use a microwave or a hair dryer, if your house is "wireless," are you out of luck? If you have immune system problems or chemical sensitivities, this could be one of the sources for your problems. A cleansing in this area would entail changing your habits – talking on the phone less, avoiding microwaves and EMF's from hair dryers, etc.

How to Do a Coffee Enema

One famous treatment clinic for cancer employs the use of coffee in enemas. Some therapists today recommend to their cancer patients that they do these enemas two times per day to keep the body detoxed. Many feel that coffee enemas shouldn't be done more than a few times each week and only after a plain salt water enema; however, certain protocols have patients having an enema twice a day while in recovery. A pinch of sea salt in the enema water will balance the fluids. This therapy has been considered unsafe by some, as enemas have come in and out of favor in different generations. It seems better to get the toxic fecal matter out of the colon using a salt water or coffee enema than it is to allow putrefying matter to stay in the colon.

Get an enema bucket or bag, a stainless steel or plastic bucket is best. Find these in the kitchen department of Target or a kitchen store. You can buy a disposable enema bag that will last several months; these are transparent, so you can observe the liquid as it leaves the bag and keep it clean.

Preparing the Coffee Enema

Use only distilled or purified water.
Find organic coffee, best if raw, but roasted can be used.
Stainless or glass pot to heat the water.

Bring 1 quart of water to a boil.
Add 4-6 T. coffee
(or put coffee in a French press and pour the boiling water over it)
Let it cool for one hour and strain the grounds from the coffee.
Pour the strained coffee into the enema bag.
Use a coat hanger to hang the enema bag on a door knob or towel holder. Moisten the tip of the enema tube with almond or castor oil and insert it into the rectum. Lie on your left side until about 1/3 of the water is retained, then roll over on the back for another 1/3, and last, roll on the right side, and retain the coffee for 10-20 minutes.
Massage your abdomen from left to right (up the left side, and then left to right just below the navel).
Try to retain for the full 20 minutes. If the urge to evacuate the bowels is very strong, try to do a warm salt water enema before you do the coffee enema the next time. If you are constipated, start with a cleansing enema using 2 quarts of warm salt water before you insert the coffee solution.
Always take probiotics to replenish your good bacteria. Some even add the good bacteria such as acidophilus to the enema water.

Cutting edge science is revealing how the gut bacteria play a huge role in your metabolism, energy, and body weight. It is certainly not the only thing that is keeping you fat (metabolic syndrome) but it is a factor worth investigating for anyone who suffers from overweight and has problems losing it and/or keeping it off.

Mice have been made obese by injecting them with bacteria from an obese human's gut. They have been able to determine that the wrong type of bacteria overgrowth in the stomach and intestinal tract are the culprit; this issue causes irrational food cravings in these mice. The two main types of bacteria of concern here are the Firmicutes and Bacteroidetes; the Firmicutes may be friendly or unfriendly, many being responsible for gut infections such as streptococcus and clostridium types of overgrowths.

In addition to the possibility of crohns and colitis symptoms and problems with weight gain, this imbalance of gut bacteria affects the brain! Probiotics can inhibit the growth of the microbiota; killing them with antibiotics is at best a temporary solution and actually causes an overgrowth of candida albicans which makes the problem much worse. It is better to avoid alcohol, and refined flours and sugars – don't give them fuel! Caprylic acid from coconut oil and oregano oil along with some pau d arco tea would be more permanent solutions.

This is a complicated problem, but there are solutions. Read David Perlmutter's book *The Brain Maker* for more helpful information about these bacteria that may be at the root of your weight, brain or nervous system problem.

Challenges for Week Six

☐ Among the many challenges for Week Six is accepting the concept that humans need to cleanse and eliminate some of the parasites and chemical waste burdening the body. Then there is the decision to go through with the cleansing process, especially the diet.

☐ Analyze your own digestion: Do you have reflux, mucus in the stools, incomplete bowel movements, constipation, or diarrhea? If so, you may need to cleanse.

☐ Do you live in the 21st century and breathe the air and drink the water that is full of chemicals, hormones, and other toxins? Then you might need to cleanse.

☐ Talk to a health professional about your lifestyle and cleansing goals. What will fit in to your life at this time?

☐ Start drinking the Master Cleanser every morning with lemon and cayenne. If you have a yeast problem, omit the maple syrup.

A final thought:

If this little book has helped you on your journey through life, it is a blessing to me. As we learn more and live more, new discoveries and insights will be revealed, and some of this information will become dated or even obsolete, but for now, it is a start. You can always visit TakeStepsToHealth.com and bettysueobrian.com

Our world changes rapidly, and speed has become expected and even demanded. Let's slow down enough to live and love our lives, ourselves, and all those with whom we share this journey. Namaste.

Betty Sue.

Where to get products and information

- Alternate Cancer Cream: www.altcancercream.com
- American College of Iridology: www.iridologycollege.org
- Andrew Weill: www.drweill.com
- Ann Wigmore Institute: www.annwigmore.org
- Aubrey Organics: www.aubrey-organics.com
- Aura Cacia Pure Aromatherapy: www.auracacia.com
- Blue Boy Herb Company: www.blueboyherbs.com
- Chakra Healing: Martin Brofman: www.healer.ch
- Dr. Bronner's Pure Castile Soaps: www.drbronner.com
- Dr. Christopher: http://schoolofnaturalhealing.com
- Eyeology Research: www.grandmedicine.com
- Essential Herb Cottage: www.essentialherbcottage.com
- Free Range Beef: www.ambergrassfedbeef.com
- Frontier Coop: www.frontiercoop.com
- Global Light Network: http://www.globallight.net
- Hylands Homeopathics: www.hylands.com
- International Iridology Practitioners' Association
- Jack Tips: www.appleaday.com
- Jeff Smith: GMO foods www.seedsofdeception.com
- Jim McDonald, Herbalist: www.herbcraft.org
- Living and Raw Foods: www.rawfoods.com
- Northeast School of Botanical Medicine: www.7song.com
- Raw Family: www.rawfamily.com
- Qigong Center for Natural Healing: www.qigong.com
- School of Natural Medicine and Farida Sharan: www.purehealth.com
- Sound Health: www.sharryedwards.com
- Tennant Institute: www.tennantinstitute.com
- Tropical Traditions: www.tropicaltraditions.com
- Uncle Harry's Natural Products: www.uncleharrys.com

- Young Living Oils: www.younglivingusa.com

Recommended Reading

- *A Course in Miracles*
- Anderson, Dr. Richard. *Arise and Shine*
- Bartlett, Richard. *Matrix Energetics*, The Science and Art of Transformation
- Braden, Greg. *The Isaiah Effect and The Divine Matrix*
- Boutenko, Victoria. *Raw Family and Green for Life*
- Brennan, Barbara. *Hands of Light and Light Emerging*
- Burroughs, Stanley. *The Master Cleanser*
- Campbell, T. Colin and Thomas M. Campbell II. *The China Study*
- Campbell, Joseph. *The Hero With a Thousand Faces*
- Capria, Fritjof. *The Tao of Physics*
- Clark, Hulda. *The Cure for All Diseases*
- Gerber, Richard. Vibrational Medicine
- Green, Glenda. *Love Without End: Jesus Speaks*
- Hawkins, David. *Power vs. Force*
- Hay, Louise. *You Can Heal Your Life*
- Jensen, Bernard. *Iridology I and II, Iridology Simplified, and Tissue Cleansing Through Bowel Management*
- Johnson, Denny. *What the Eye Reveals*
- Myss, Caroline. *Anatomy of the Spirit and The Creation of Health*
- O'Brian, Betty and Jack Tips. *Causations: Using Sclerology to Clarify Iridology*
- O'Brian, Betty. *Going Green...with Smoothies*
- Primack, Jeff and Anne Jinnett. *Smoothie Formulas: 54 Specific Recipes for 3hpBlending.* Available at www.qigong.com
- Sharan, Farida. *Herbs of Grace*
- Starr, Mark, M.D. *Type II Hypothyroidism*
- Tennant, Jerry. *Healing is Voltage*
- Yogananda, Paramhansa. *Autobiography of a Yogi*
- Young, Robert. *The pH Miracle, The pH Miracle for Diabetes*
- Tips, Jack. *The Pro-Vita! Plan for Optimal Nutrition*

A Few More Recipes

My favorite Warming, Vegetarian Soups and Cool Salads that are Hearty and Filling:

Kitcheree (Mung Bean Soup)[38]

Add 1/2 cup of mung beans to 10-12 cups of filtered water.

Boil the mung beans with 3/4 c. brown basmati rice first for about 10 minutes.

While that is boiling, sauté the following in a little extra virgin coconut oil or olive oil:

> 1 finely chopped onion,
>
> 10 cloves of sliced or chopped garlic
>
> 2- 3 T. peeled and chopped ginger root
>
> 1 tsp. turmeric,
>
> 1/2 tsp. ground black pepper
>
> 1/ tsp. crushed red chili flakes
>
> 1/2 tsp. cumin

Add vegetables; cover and boil gently 30 minutes.

Then add 1 or 2 cups of any chopped vegetables, carrots, Swiss chard, asparagus, celery, etc.

Add a little Braggs Liquid Aminos towards the end and top with yogurt.

Garden Vegetable Soup

1 cup chopped celery

1 1/2 cup sliced, organic carrots

1 1/2 cup chopped onions

1 1/2 cup frozen peas

1/3 cup fresh parsley

1 T. fresh rosemary

3-4 cloves chopped garlic

6 cups organic V8 juice or 6 tomatoes chopped and 4 cups veggie broth

1 T. Celtic sea salt

T. Pepper

Bay Leaves

---

[38] Meredith Wright, Kundalini Yoga Center of Houma, LA

Add all ingredients, and then add water to equal about 1 – 1 1/2 gallons. Simmer but do not overcook.

Fiesta Chopped Salad

2 tomatoes, chopped

1 cucumber, peeled and chopped

1 each red, green, yellow bell pepper, chopped

1 small red onion, chopped 1 can diced green chilies

14 c. fresh cilantro, chopped 3 T. salsa

2 Tbs. Fresh-squeezed lemon juice

1/2 Tbs. garlic, minced 1/4 tsp. pepper

1/4 tsp. sea salt

1/4 tsp. ground cumin

Combine all ingredients and chill for one hour. Serve on a bed of lettuce or with sprouted tortilla chips.

Black Beans with a Hint of Citrus

4 cups dried black beans (preferably organic)

1 large carrot, chopped fine

3 quarts water

2-3 sprigs parsley

3 bay leaves

2 Tbsp. extra virgin olive oil 2 tsp. sea salt

2 chopped peppers (I use one bell pepper and 1/2 jalapeno)

1 small onion, chopped

2 Tbsp. chili powder

1 T. crushed cumin seed

4 cloves fresh garlic, chopped small 1/3 cup fresh squeezed orange juice

Soak the beans overnight. Add the carrot and onion, salt and pepper, and simmer until beans are soft.

Sauté the rest of the ingredients in the olive oil for 3-5 minutes and add to the beans. Let simmer for 20 more minutes.

Then add the orange juice and the garlic. Cover with a lid and cook for 10 more minutes. Enjoy over rice or plain as a soup with organic corn chips!

Killer Kale

Organic kale

1 t. Garlic, minced finely

1 t. Celtic sea salt

T. EV olive oil

Stir for 3-5 minutes. Massage the leaves carefully to release the nutrients. Serve in 1-2 hours. Add a little Braggs Aminos if you need extra flavor

Yogi Tea or Chai[39]

Fill a medium pot with 2 quarts of filtered water.

Add 8 cinnamon sticks, 1 heaping tablespoon of cardamom seeds, 1/2 tablespoon of whole cloves, 1/2 tablespoon of black peppercorns and 5 slices of fresh ginger root.

Boil 30 minutes.

Reduce heat and simmer on a low flame for 2 hours. Add water as necessary.

Remove from heat and let tea sit all night. In the morning, strain and store in fridge.

After heating the tea the next day, add 1-2 teabags of black tea. Steep one minute. The black tea is an important healing catalyst in the tea.

You might add raw milk and honey to taste. Based upon the teachings in this book, try to learn to drink it without the milk, as we know how the mucus in dairy disagrees with most human bodies.

---

[39] Guru Dev Kaur Khalsa, www.earthclinic.com/Remedies/yogitea

Getting Serious About Your Smoothies

"Do I have to Drink them?" Yes, smoothies are a necessary part of your daily routine for many reasons:

- Pollution
- Pour Assimilation
- Bad Digestion
- Poor Chewing
- Lack of desire to eat so many fruits or vegetables

A good fruit and veggie smoothie will give you the PHYTONUTRIENTS or PHYTO CHEMICALS you might need in a whole day. If you add enough ingredients to your morning smoothie, you won't get hungry for junk food because your cells will be SINGING out loud. Your body will be healing so fast when you start a daily regimen of blended smoothies. At first, you might want to rebel against some of the ingredients, but you will end up thanking me for suggesting that you try some of these simple drinks.

In this book, I gave you some simple recipes, but now I want to introduce you to the concept of blending smoothies with a Vita Mix or other powerful blender. If you can't get one right now, use what you have, but the more you can micronize the food, the more you will absorb from it. So here, I am offering you a few recipes from another of my books *Going Green; The Smoothie Way*, but you might want to invent your own, too. Just blend and enjoy.

Avocado/Coconut Shake

Avocado without the skin and seed
1/2 pineapple including the stem
T. flaked organic coconut or grated fresh coconut 1 carrot
2 cups. water and 5 ice cubes
1/4 t. green stevia if desired

Liver Cleansing Dynamite

1 whole apple (including seeds)
peeled lemon (including the white membrane)
1 unpeeled organic cucumber (peel if not organic)
1/2 beet
Quarter size piece of peeled ginger
2 Cups Water

This drink is the perfect blend of sweet and sour; it tastes yummy.

Energy Smoothie

1/2 cup blueberries 1/2 cup blackberries 5-8 strawberries 2 stalks celery
1 carrot
1 cup spinach
1/2 red bell pepper 2 cups water
Pinch of stevia or 1 t. agave nectar

Citrus Delight Parasite Drink – every day for 7-10 days

1 whole orange
1 whole grapefruit
1/2 t. turmeric
1/2 t. cinnamon
1/4 t. cayenne
1 T. flax or hemp seeds
2 cups water
*Optional but worth it: 2 cloves garlic
Blend and Enjoy.

About the Author

Traditional Naturopath and Nutrition Consultant Betty Sue O'Brian studied dietetics as an undergraduate at the University of Southern Mississippi and applied her education to raise a "natural family." In 1980, she co-founded the Hattiesburg, MS, Natural Foods Cooperative. With an intense interest in natural health, she began a Shaklee Vitamin business in her home.

In 1982, she met Jeanette Shaw, an iridologist and herbalist who helped her infant survive an allergy to soy-based formulas by supplying fresh, raw goat's milk from her farm. Ten years later Jeanette helped her through Chronic Fatigue and a systemic yeast infection. Those two incidences inspired the author to become an herbalist and to study natural medicine more deeply.

Betty Sue is now a naturopath with a Natural Physicians degree (one whose path is the natural way), a certified Master Sclerologist, a diplomat instructor for the International Iridology Practitioners' Association, and an herbalist with degrees from the School of Natural Medicine in Boulder, Colorado. She has studied and attended classes at the Ann Wigmore Institute and the International Sclerology Institute, and taken courses from Dr. Bernard Jensen, Dr. Jack Tips, Dr. Farida Sharan, Dr. Danielle LoRito, Master Herbalist Darrell Martin and others from around the world. She is the Past President of the International Iridology Practitioners' Association

This quote from the New Testament inspires her studies of the eye. The physician Luke says, "Your eye is the lamp of your body; when your eye is not sound, your body is full of darkness. Therefore, be careful lest the light in you be darkness. If then your whole body is full of light, having no part dark, it will be wholly bright, as when a lamp with its rays gives you light." -Luke 11:33

Please find Betty Sue on Facebook as "Betty Sue Says", send an email to betty.obrian@gmail.com, or visit her websites at www.bettysueobrian.com, iridologyacademy.org, and takestepstohealth.com.

Other Books by Betty Sue O'Brian

These books are all available on Amazon.

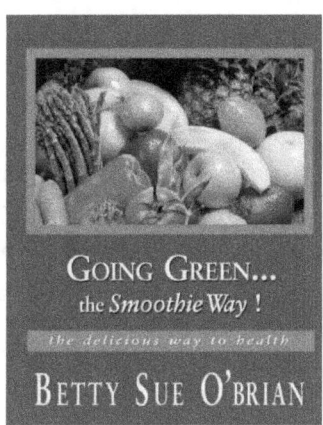

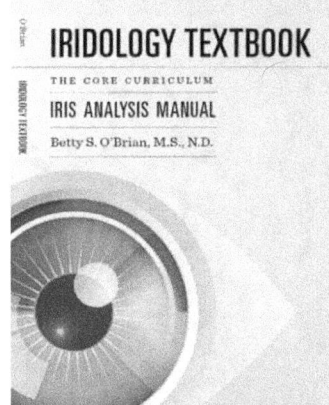

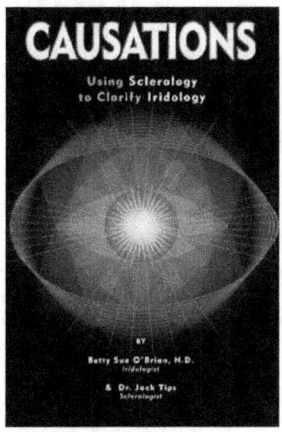